INSTITUTIONAL CARE AND THE MENTALLY HANDICAPPED

The Mental Handicap Hospital

Institutional Care and the Mentally Handicapped

The Mental Handicap Hospital

ANDY ALASZEWSKI, PhD
Senior Lecturer, Department of Social Policy
and Professional Studies, University of Hull

CROOM HELM
London • Sydney • Dover, New Hampshire

43540

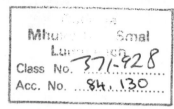
Croom Helm Ltd, Provident House, Burrell Row,
Beckenham, Kent BR3 1AT
Croom Helm Australia Pty Ltd, Suite 4, 6th Floor,
64-76 Kippax Street, Surry Hills, NSW 2010, Australia

British Library Cataloguing in Publication Data

Alaszewski, Andy
    Institutional care and the mentally handicapped:
    the mental handicap hospital.
    1. Psychiatric hospitals − England
    I. Title
    362.3'85'0942   RC450.G7
    ISBN 0-7099-0564-5

Croom Helm, 51 Washington Street, Dover,
New Hampshire 03820, USA

Library of Congress Cataloging in Publication Data

Alaszewski, Andy.
    Institutional care and the mentally handicapped.

    Originally presented as author's thesis (Ph.D.−
University of Cambridge).
    Bibliography: p.
    Includes index.
    1. Mental retardation facilities−Great Britain.
2. Jane Eagle Hospital−Case studies. 3. Mental
retardation facilities−Great Britain−Administration.
4. Mentally handicapped−Institutional care−Great
Britain. 5. Handicapped−Functional assessment.
I. Jane Eagle Hospital. II. Title. [DNLM: 1. Hospitals,
Psychiatric−organization & administration−Great
Britain. 2. Mental Health Services−organization &
administration−Great Britain. 3. Patients−classification.
WM 30 A3236i]
HV3008.G7A72   1986   362.2'1'0941   85-22025
ISBN 0-7099-0564-5

Printed and bound in Great Britain
by Billing & Sons Limited, Worcester.

CONTENTS

TABLES AND DIAGRAMS

Tables and Diagrams

Tables and Diagrams

ACKNOWLEDGEMENTS

I received a research studentship from the Social Science Research Council for the research on which this book is based. The Social and Political Studies Committee of the Faculty of Economics and Politics at the University of Cambridge provided the academic support and supervision for the project. Gilbert Lewis of the Department of Social Anthropology acted as my supervisor. He provided me with considerable support during the difficult periods and improved my writing style. He gave me the confidence I needed to complete my research.

I received both information and friendship from the nurses at the Jane Eagle Hospital. I have tried not to take their ideas and actions out of context.

One nurse in particular was a considerable source of support and advice during the research, my wife, Helen. Few researchers can have had the opportunity to talk so readily and easily to such a sympathetic and insightful informant. Her judgement has always been faultless.

Petrina Atkinson helped with the preparation of the camera ready copy of this book. She was extremely patient and good humoured during this difficult final stage of the preparation of the book.

Gill Manthorpe made helpful comments on the final version of this book.

For Helen

PREFACE

     This book is based on a dissertation that was accepted by the University of Cambridge for the degree of Doctor of Philosophy in 1981. The only major alteration I have made to the dissertation is to write a new introductory chapter outlining the history of institutions and to incorporate an article on staff training as Chapter Six. I wrote my dissertation as a book rather than an academic monograph and on rereading I felt it was suitable for publication and I hope that the readers of this book will agree with me.
     The research was conducted in the mid-seventies. Important changes have occurred in the last decade. In some ways this book is a historical record of institutions at one stage of their development. The institution I researched no longer exists. The buildings are still there but most of the staff and patients I worked with have left. In this book I develop a general theory of institutions based on my research in one particular institution. Therefore my analysis is not limited to a particular time.
     The book is divided into four parts. In Part One, I set the scene for my analysis by examining the development and history of institutions (Chapter One) and describing the methods I used in my study (Chapter Two). In the second part, (Chapters Three to Five) I examine the structure of ideas in one institution and I discuss various aspects of the different systems of classification. In the third part, I examine the structure of social action in the institution. I examine the ways in which the institution reproduced itself through nurse training, (Chapter Six), the ways in which the institution structures

1

social activities   such as eating   (Chapter Seven)
and the   strategies of control in   the institution
(Chapter   Eight).   The   final part   contains   one
chapter, in   which I examine information   my study
provides about the   general nature of   institutions
in contemporary society.

CHAPTER 1
THE INSTITUTION

1.1 INTRODUCTION

The bulk of this book is devoted to a study
of one specific institution, a Mental Handicap
Hospital, which I refer to as the Jane Eagle
Hospital. As I want this case study to illustrate
the characteristics of institutions, I shall in
this chapter place my study into the context of
the historical development of institutions. I am
concerned to identify the unique distinguishing
features of institutions as a basis of my
subsequent discussion of these features in one
specific institution. In the first section I
shall provide a preliminary definition of the
institution, in the second I shall discuss the
emergence of the modern institution at the
beginning of the 19th Century, in the third
section I shall discuss the development of Mental
Deficiency Colonies at the beginning of the 20th
Century and in the fourth and final section I
shall consider alternatives to institutions and
the information they provide about the nature of
institutions.

1.2 THE INSTITUTION: A PRELIMINARY DEFINITION

Definitions of institutions are fairly rare,
it is usually accepted that everyone knows what an
institution is.
Jones and Fowles provide a relatively bland
definition of an institution as "any long-term
provision of a highly-organised kind on a
residential basis with the expressed aims of
"care", "treatment" or "custody"" (Jones and
Fowles: 1984, p.207). This is an inclusive rather

than an exclusive definition and is not helpful in identifying and explaining the characteristics of institutions. A useful starting point is Goffman's definition of a total institution as "a place of residence and work where a large number of like-situated individuals, cut off from the wider society for an appreciable period of time, together lead an enclosed, formally administered round of life" (Goffman: 1968, p.xiii). Some of the features stressed by Goffman: size, isolation and totality, refer only to some institutions. The common features of institutions are implicit in the "formally administered round of life". The inmate's life is administered by staff.

Street, Vinter and Perrow (1966) extended Goffman's definition. They suggested that total institutions are a form of "people-changing organization". They utilized Janowitz's definition of these organisations as "institutions that have the goal of changing human personality and human values so that their clients can participate effectively in the larger society" (Street, Vinter and Perrow: 1966, p.v). They laid great stress on the formal goals of the institution which they defined as the goals of the senior personnel. They identified three types of people-changing organisations : custodial, re-educative and therapeutic.

Street, Vinter and Perrow's approach assumed that the senior personnel's objectives were shared by other staff, and this in turn affected their attitude to the inmates.

> The key hypothesis here is that variations in organizational goals are accompanied by variations in staff's sets of beliefs about the inmates - what they are like and what must be done to change them.
> (Street, Vinter and Perrow: 1966, p.142)

Their own evidence suggested systematic variation between staff attitudes to inmates.

> More highly educated staff members scored higher on understanding and lower on discipline than other staff members in every organizational setting, but the institutional differences held up within categories of educational levels.
> (Street, Vinter and Perrow: 1966, p.145)

4

Street, Vinter and Perrow implicitly provided an alternative definition of institutions when they asserted that "the basic productive task of the juvenile institution, like that of all people-changing organizations, lies in structuring social relations between staff and inmates" (Street, Vinter and Perrow: 1966, p.151). All institutions share one feature, one group of people, the inmates, are dependent on another, the staff, for some or all of the basic necessities of life, such as food and clothing. There exists between inmates and staff an unequal dependence relationship. This contrasts strongly with relationships outside the institution where relations of dependency are based on ties of kinship. Otherwise the norm of relationships is equality and independence, and this is epitomised in the contract - an agreement voluntarily established between formally independent and equal individuals. If this overall definition is accepted then a typology of institutions can be developed, based on the official reasons for the dependency, e.g. institutions in which dependency is imposed as a punishment (prisons), institutions in whch dependency is accepted as a means toward an end (hospitals for acute physical illness) and institutions coping with intrinsic dependency (hospitals for the mentally handicapped). These would be ideal types. In practice any given institution could be classified in a variety of ways and there could be disagreement amongst the participants about the cause of dependency.

1.3   THE ORIGINS AND STRUCTURE OF MODERN INSTITUTIONS

The development of industrial society was marked by a transformation of the productive, ideological and political structures of society resulting in qualitative changes in the pattern of social and economic relations.

One way of describing this change was as a shift from relations based on social status, where individual rights and obligations were defined by social status ascribed at birth, to relations based on contract in which individual rights and obligations were defined by agreement as expressed in various forms of contracts (Maine : 1866). Maine argued that contractual relations could never completely replace status relations as there

would always remain individuals excluded from relations which arise from "the free agreement of individuals", i.e. children, orphans and lunatics who are "subject to extrinsic control on the single ground that they do not posses the faculty of forming a judgement on their own interests" (Maine: 1866, pp.169-170).
One aspect of the transformation was the emergence of the modern institution. Social historians have shown that institutional life was practically unknown in pre-industrial society (Laslett: 1965, p.11).
In the United States the rapid development of institutions in the early 19th Century has been described by Rothman.

> The question this book addresses can be
> put very succinctly: why did Americans
> in the Jacksonian era suddenly begin to
> construct and support institutions for
> deviant and dependent members of the
> community? ... Here was a revolution
> in social practices ... The few
> institutions that existed in the
> eighteenth century were clearly places
> of last resort. Americans in the
> Jacksonian period reversed these
> practices. Institutions became places
> of first resort. (Rothman: 1971,
> p.xii)

Rothman showed how the shift from small scale relatively stable communities to large scale communities with a large mobile population of immigrants spelt the end of workhouses and other traditional forms of public assistance as informal methods of community self-help and created the conditions for the large scale Institutions. However, he also argued that increased problems of social control associated with industrialisation, urbanisation and increased migration did not in themselves account for the form and nature of the new institutions. They were based on and involved a new conception of society. They were attempts to create model societies within society. They can be seen as zones of dependency amongst independent individuals.
In England the foundation of the new institutions was closely associated with the first investigations and reports of traditional forms of

6

social control and care. Dependency in its
various forms exerted a considerable pull on the
contemporary imagination. Prisons, workhouses and
hospitals all attracted attention.

However special interest was devoted to the
madness and madhouses. Tuke's description of the
Retreat in York published in 1813 (Tuke: 1813) was
followed by the Report of the House of Commons
Select Committee on Madhouses (1815). The two
reports were interrelated (Tuke: 1964). The
exposure of conditions at York Asylum led to the
establishment of the Select Committee that exposed
the conditions of the mad living in Bethlem,
private madhouses and local workhouses.

Both Tuke and the Select Committee were
concerned with the treatment of the mad and with
improving this treatment. This involved separating
the mad from other types of dependants (and by
implication madness from other forms of
dependency) and developing special institutions
for the mad. Tuke furthered this objective by
providing and describing a model institution and
describing how it could provide specialist or
moral treatment through a special staff:inmate
relationship and by creating a special rhythm of
life. The Select Committee argued that
traditional facilities were unsuitable for the
treatment of the mad and madness (The Select
Committee on Madhouses: 1815, p.2).

Although the Select Committee Reports did not
immediately achieve their objective, they started
a campaign that eventually resulted in a
specialist legislative and institutional framework
for the mad (Jones: 1972).

These early institutions shared three
distinctive characteristics: special architecture,
a concern with proper classification and a
distinctive structure of activities. I shall
discuss each of these characteristics in turn.

Special Architecture

Traditional facilities such as private
madhouses, workhouses or prisons were not usually
purpose-built. They were established in and made
use of existing buildings. Prisoners were often
held in castles, whereas madhouses used domestic
houses. The reformers were critical of the use of
existing buildings. For example the Select
Committee on Madhouses described existing
madhouses in the following way:

> in a few of them the arrangement is good..
> as the contracted size of the houses,
> and the small extent of the ground
> attached to them, will admit; and that
> the treatment of the inhabitants in
> them has been kind and proper; - but it
> is in proof, that there is just and
> great cause of complaint against by far
> the greater part of the houses of this
> description, which have hardly, in any
> instance, been built for the purpose, and
> are incapable of being conveniently
> adapted to it. (Report of the Committee
> on Madhouses: 1815, p.2)

The Select Committee was so concerned about
the inadequacy of existing buildings that it
obtained and made public the plans for a model
asylum.

> Your Committee, impressed with the
> inadequacy of the Buildings for the
> reception of Insane Persons throughout
> England, obtained from an Architect,
> who has given great attention to this
> subject, and who has been employed to
> make designs for an Asylum for the
> West Riding of York, Plans with Estimates,
> which they think may be useful to the
> public, especially in counties where there
> may be a disposition to erect houses for
> the reception of Insane Persons. (Report
> of the Committee on Madhouses: 1815,
> pp.5-6)

Similarly the first substantive chapter in
Tuke's description of the Retreat was devoted to
an account of the grounds and of the house (Tuke:
1964, pp.92-107).

The reformers at the beginning of the 19th
Century were optimistic about the new
Institutions as places of care and treatment.
However as the century progressed this optimism
was replaced by pessimism and the asylums grew in
size and capacity (See Table 1.1). As Scull
(1979) has argued, they become warehouses of the
insane.

Whereas the early asylums were relatively
small scale, the Retreat was initially designed
for 30 patients, the later asylums were large

Table 1.1 Growth of the Asylum System in England and Wales in the Nineteenth Century.

Date	Number of Asylums	Average Size
1 Jan 1827	9	116.0
1 Jan 1850	24	297.5
1 Jan 1860	41	386.7
1 Jan 1870	51	548.6
1 Jan 1880	61	657.2
1 Jan 1890	66	802.1

(Source - Scull: 1979, p.198)

scale. Colney Hatch, the Middlesex Asylum opened in 1851, was designed for 1000 patients. The increasing scale of asylums necessitated special designs and purpose built facilities. For example a competition was held for the design of buildings for Colney Hatch and the contract was placed with a major building company. The construction involved over 1000 workmen, and 10 million bricks were made and laid (Hunter and MacAlpine: 1974, pp.21-25). The new institutional architecture tended to appear very grand and impressive from the outside but internally to be barren. Colney Hatch was described by one contemporary visitor in the following way:

> Its facade, of nearly a third of a mile, is
>   broken at intervals by Italian campaniles
>   and cupolas, and the whole aspect of the
>   exterior leads the visitor to expect
>   an interior of commensurate pretensions.
>   He no sooner crosses the threshold,
>   however, than the scene changes. As he
>   passes along the corridor, which runs
>   from end to end of the building, he is
>   oppressed with gloom ... (quoted in Scull:
>   1979, p.196)

Scull suggests that the architectural harmony of Colney Hatch was atypical as most asylums grew rather haphazardly, nevertheless they were housed in distinctive and unmistakable buildings.

Other types of institutions also developed their own distinctive institutional architecture. Rothman has shown that the architecture of prisons in the U.S.A. at the end of the Eighteenth Century "still commonly followed the model of the

household" and that a widely copied prison, Walnut
Street jail, resembled an ordinary, if somewhat
large, frame house, indistinguishable from other
sizeable dwellings" (Rothman: 1971, p.90). In
contrast the new prisons of the 1820's were
distinctive purpose built structures in which few
costs were spared to achieve the reformers'
blueprints (Rothman: 1971, pp.94-101).

Proper Classification of Inmates

The special architecture of the new
institutions served a variety of different
functions. For example the reformers at the
beginning of the Nineteenth Century saw special
buildings as a way of improving patient care and
treatment, by the end of the century the emphasis
had shifted to economy and cost minimisation.
However underlying these disparate concerns was a
common and persisting interest in the
classification of inmates.

The reformers criticised traditional
facilities because they mixed different sorts of
people. They allowed the normal and abnormal to
mix and they allowed different types of abnormal
people to mix. The special architecture was
designed to segregate the normal from the abnormal
and to separate different sorts and classes of
abnormal people.

The concern to separate and correctly
allocate the mad is evident in the Committee on
Madhouses concern about the implementation of
permissive legislation for the construction of
asylums:

> in order to prevent the intolerable evil of
> these unhappy persons being imprisoned in
> gaols or in parish workhouses, or
> permitted to wander about the country in a
> state of total helplessness and neglect;
> in the former case, to the great annoyance
> of other prisoners or poor, as well as
> unnecessary restraint and suffering to
> themselves; and in the latter to the
> great danger of their doing mischief to
> others or to themselves. (Report of the
> Committee on Madhouses: 1815, p.6)

Inside the asylum the committee was concerned
about the mixing of different sorts of patients
especially:

> The mixing of Patients who are outrageous,
> with those who are quiet and inoffensive;
> and those who are insensible to the call
> of nature, with those who are cleanly.
> (Report of the Committee on Madhouses:
> 1815, p.3)

The link between architecture and
classification is clear in Tuke's description of
the Retreat. Although he saw the Retreat as a
model, he stressed that each asylum would have to
have its own design adapted to its own particular
classification of patients:

> It is not ... to be supposed that the
> Retreat ... should be a perfect model for
> establishments of this kind ... Indeed,
> it is hardly probable, as the class of
> persons, both as to rank and disease,
> in different establishments, must be
> various, that the arrangements in any one,
> can be precisely followed in another.
> (Tuke: 1964, p.104)

Tuke saw the proper classification of
patients in the Retreat as an essential part of
the care and treatment of the patients:

> in all houses established for the reception
> of the insane, the general comfort of
> the patients ought to be considered; and
> those who are violent, require to be
> separated from the more tranquil, and to
> be prevented, by some means, from
> offensive conduct, 'towards their fellow-
> sufferers. Hence, the patients are
> arranged into classes, as much as may be,
> according to the degree in which they
> approach to rational or orderly conduct.
> (Tuke: 1964, p.141)

In the larger Victorian asylums proper
classification was achieved through the separation
of different classes of patients into different
wards. For example the 1000 patients at Colney
Hatch Asylum were grouped into wards "numbered
1-14 for men, 15-32 for women and built as long
galleries sleeping 30-40 patients in a row of
small single rooms with a 4-5 bedded dormitory in
the centre on one side" (Hunter and MacAlpine:

1974, p.27-28). The overt purpose of the classification had altered from care and treatment of the patients to management and control as is clear from Granville's observations that

> the classification generally made is for
> the purpose of shelving cases; that is to
> say, practically it has that effect ... in
> consequence of the treatment not being
> personal, but simply a treatment in
> classes, there is a tendency to make whole
> classes sink down into a sort of chronic
> state ... I think they come under a sort
> of routine discipline which ends in their
> passing into a state of dementia.
> (quoted in Scull: 1979, p.200)

Institutional Routine
    The distinctive classification of patients into units or wards was associated with a special institutional organisation of inmates' activities. In the Retreat, the activities of everyday life were organised as part of treatment of the patients. Patients were assessed in terms of their ability to perform these activities:

> They (patients) quickly perceive, or if
> not, they are informed on the first
> occasion, that their treatment depends,
> in general measure, upon their conduct.
> (Tuke: 1964, p.141)

One important indicator of the patients' sanity was the ways in which they ate. The sanest patients ate at the family meals and the maddest had to be force fed, with various gradations of madness in between (Tuke: 1964, pp.168-171). The organisation of employment formed an important part of the treatment:

> Of all the modes by which the patients may
> be induced to restrain themselves,
> regular employment is perhaps the most
> generally efficacious; and those kinds
> of employment are doubtless to be
> preferred, both on a moral and physical
> account, which are accompanied by
> considerable bodily action; that are
> most agreeable to the patient, and which
> are the most opposite to the illusions of

his disease. (Tuke: 1964, p.156)

Perhaps the most dramatic examples of
institutional regulation of inmate activities can
be found in American prisons in the 1820's.
Tocqueville and Beaumont described the nature of
life in contemporary prisons in the following
way:

> We have no doubt but that the habits of
> order to which the prisoner is subjected
> for several years ... the obedience of
> every moment to inflexible rules, the
> regularity of a uniform life, in a word,
> all the circumstances belonging to this
> severe system, are calculated to produce
> a deep impression upon his mind.
> (cited in Rothman: 1971, p.103)

The organisation of prisoners' activities
even affected the way prisoners walked. A special
form of walk was invented for the movement of
prisoners in the new prisons:

> Regimentation became the standard mode of
> prison life. Convicts did not walk from
> place to place; rather, they went in
> close order and single file, each looking
> over the shoulder of the man in front,
> faces inclined to the right, feet moving
> in unison, in lockstep. The lockstep
> became the trademark of American prisons
> in these years, a curious combination of
> march and shuffle that remained standard
> procedure well into the 1930's.
> (Rothman: 1971, pp.105-106)

Comment
Although 19th Century institutions were
established for diverse purposes and with diverse
motives, they shared certain common features. They
did not use existing buildings but were
established in distinctive purpose built
facilities. These buildings separated the inmates
from the rest of society and inside the
institution provided for the separation of
different classes of inmates. The activities of
inmates inside the institution was consciously
planned and structured in a distinctive routine or
regime.

13

1.4   THE MENTAL DEFICIENCY COLONY

The development of special institutional facilities for mentally handicapped people is a relatively recent development. At the beginning of the 19th Century idiots and imbeciles were not recognised by the reformers as a distinctive group with special needs. In the 1850's and 60's the situation changed and a number of specialist institutions were opened such as the Northern Counties Asylum for Idiots and Imbeciles in Lancaster (Jones: 1972, p.182). These institutions were isolated local ventures. In 1881 a census of idiots in public institutions identified 29,452. Most of these were in Poor Law Institutions. Only 3% were in special Idiots' Asylums (Jones: 1972, p.183). In 1914 there were still only 6 special institutions with 2,040 idiots (Commissioners in Lunacy: 1914, p.14).

In 1904 the government appointed a Royal Commission to investigate the Care and Control of the Feeble-Minded. The Royal Commission reported in 1908 and it recommended the establishment of a special legal and administrative structure to care for and control mental defectives. The Commission recommended that each local authority establish an institution or colony as the basis of its services. The main recommendations of the Commission formed the basis of the 1913 Mental Deficiency Act. However, because of the 1st World War and the limitations on local authority expenditure, little progress was made in implementing the provisions of the Act.

In 1924 a Mental Deficiency Committee was established to consider the education and care of mental defectives. This Committee reported in 1929. It endorsed the findings of the 1904 Royal Commission and argued for the rapid expansion of institutional provision. The Committee identified mental defectives as a problem group of dependants who lived in the community:

> the members composing a community may be broadly divided into two groups. First, there are those whose mentality is such as to allow of the independent performance of their duties in some social situation in a reasonably satisfactory and efficient manner. Secondly, there are those whose mentality is such as to render such

> independent and efficient adaptation
> impossible, and who consequently need some
> form of special surroundings or some
> degree of external assistance, control
> or supervision. (Within this second
> category the committee identified mental
> defectives as one sub-class as) Persons
> whose incapacity is due to their minds
> having failed to reach what may be
> termed a normal degree of development.
> (Report of the Mental Deficiency
> Committee: 1929, Part 1, para.14)

Following the Report of the Committee there
was a rapid expansion of specialised institutional
provision (See Table 1.2) (For a fuller account
of these developments see Ayer and Alaszewski:
1984, pp.4-18). The development of specialist
institutional facilities for mentally defective
people had the same characteristics as the general
expansion of other institutions in the 19th
Century. There were, in the various official
reports, criticisms of existing facilities
associated with a concern with the proper design
and construction of institutions and the control
of the daily activities of defectives.

Table 1.2 Growth of Mental Deficiency System 1924
to 1954

Date	Total in Institutions
1924	17,104
1929	24,207
1934	35,794
1939	46,054
1944	51,214
1949	54,887
1954	55,984
Target(Wood Committee)	100,000

(Source Rooff: 1957, p.169)

The Special Design of Colonies

As the bulk of contemporary facilities for mental defectives were in workhouses, the 1904 Royal Commission started its investigation by considering the quality of care and control of mental defectives in workhouses. The Commission received conflicting evidence. Those concerned with workhouses felt they provided a reasonable quality of service. Others, especially medical experts, felt workhouses were inadequate and specialist facilities were needed. The Royal Commission came down on the side of the critics of the workhouses. They felt that in the workhouses:

> there are special arrangements, here and
> there, for the care of the mentally
> defective ... but ... as a whole, the
> accommodation now provided for these
> persons is insufficient, unsatisfactory,
> and unsuitable. (Report of the Royal
> Commission on the Care and Control of the
> Feeble Minded: 1908, para.112)

The Royal Commission advocated the development of special institutions or colonies as they felt that "the colony system is likely to produce the best moral and economic results" (para. 261). The Commission sent a deputation to the United States "in order to see the more remarkable American Institutions" (para.850). The Commission was so impressed with these American colonies that they appended to their main report a full account of the visit and the designs of various colonies. In England, the only suitable model, was the Darenth Institutions developed by the Metropolitan Asylum Board for the care of mental defectives from London. It was also commended by the Commission.

> The Darenth institutions may be said in some
> measure to represent the first experiment
> of uniting in one colony improvable
> children, young persons over sixteen, and
> adults, an experiment which is not yet
> fully made, but is a process of develop-
> ment... Altogether there are about 1,900
> persons, excluding the staff. About 500
> of these, under sixteen, are in the
> schools; another 400 helpless and hopeless

cases are in the pavilions, and in the
industrial colony there are about 1,053.
(Report of the Royal Commission on the
Care and Control of the Feeble-Minded:
1908, para.257)

The Royal Commission did not provide a
detailed blueprint for the new colonies. It was
more concerned with establishing the case for
broad legal and administrative charges. The 1929
Committee, in contrast, could take this legal and
administrative framework for granted and was able
to discuss the new institutions in more detail,
although it was also still concerned to establish
the case for purpose built colonies over Poor
Law Institutions.

Some of us have had the opportunity of
comparing the happiness, the condition,
and the behaviour of patients in a modern
colony for defectives with that of
defectives in small groups in ordinary
Poor Law Institutions, and we have no
doubt whatever that the life of the
colony ensures the greater measure of
health, happiness, contentment and useful
employment. (Report of the Mental
Deficiency Committee: 1929, Part III,
para.18)

The Committee strongly advocated village
colonies, in which the patients were housed in
villas clustered around a central administrative
block:

There is a concensus (sic) of opinion
amongst those in a position to judge,
that, so far as the central institution
is concerned, any new provision for
defectives, should be made in village
Colonies. By this method proper
classification in small units, varied
trades and industries, suitably graded
schools, economic maintenance, specialist
medical attention, hospital facilities,
adequate training of staff and
opportunities for research can all be
secured. (Report of the Mental Deficiency
Committee: 1929, Part III, para.70)

The Committee was concerned about the costs of these new colonies so they suggested a local authority could spread the cost of buying the site and gradually developing a full-scale colony:

> It may perhaps be convenient, when planning an institution, to provide in the first instance for only one or two grades of defectives, say the young and trainable cases, and gradually to extend, but it must not be forgotten that the Act has laid on the Authorities the duty of providing for all ages, grades and types of defect. Consequently it is essential that the estate purchased and the ultimate plans for its development should provide not only for those young and trainable cases, but also for the low grade cases, both children and adults, for the higher grade adults, both stable and unstable, for some types of older defectives; for the immoral, and for those who have been in prisons. (Report of the Mental Deficiency Committee: 1929, Part III, para.74)

The Committee specified that a full colony should have:

> Apart from the separate villas for each group, a central administrative block, a properly arranged school and workshops for the various trades, the colony, when fully developed, should certainly include a small hospital block on modern lines, a farm with the requisite farm buildings, a large recreation hall, sufficient playing fields, cottages for married attendants, and a nurses' home. (Report of the Mental Deficiency Committee: 1929, Part III, para.73)

The central body responsible for mental defectives, The Board of Control, was so concerned about the design of institutions that it appointed a special Departmental Committee:

> to consider and report what are the essential stuctural requirements of a complete colony for mental defectives

> of all types . (Report of
> the Committee on the Constuction
> of Colonies: 1931, para.1)

This Committee produced a comprehensive
report on the design of colonies and included an
appendix with 10 separate designs from which local
committees could choose, and details of the most
economic methods of construction.

The Proper Classification of Patients

The concern with the proper classification of
defectives formed a recurrent theme in the
official reports. The 1904 Royal Commission
criticised existing Poor Law facilities for the
mentally defective because they were not suited to
a proper classification of defectives and mixed
together different types of defectives:

> if the Poor Law administration of the
> country were to be expanded to meet the
> actual needs of mentally defective
> persons, very great changes would have to
> be made in its whole structure. The
> system of classification, so far as it
> affects this class, would have to be
> entirely revised. That intermingling (of
> different types of defectives) to which in
> different processes many witnesses
> referred would have to come to an end.
> (Report of the Royal Commission on the
> Care and Control of the Feeble-Minded:
> 1908, para.119)

One of the main features of the large
American colonies, that impressed the members of
the Commission during their American visit, was
their system of classification. Members of the
Commission were:

> impressed by the large size of American
> institutions some of which contained from
> 500 to 2,000 inmates. This seems to them
> to secure proper classification, the
> general plan being that each institution
> contains three departments, and it is
> perfectly easy to transfer an inmate from
> one to the other. These departments are,
> the Custodial for the lowest grade (i.e.
> idiots), the school for the higher grade

19

> children, and the industrial for the
> higher grade adults. (Report of the Royal
> Commission on the Care and Control of the
> Feeble-Minded:1908, para.854)

A concern with the proper classification of mental defectives also formed a recurrent theme in the Report of the Mental Deficiency Committee. It was concerned with classification in the sense of separating the normal from the abnormal. For example it felt that normal school children should be protected from:

> children of very low grade, those whose
> presence would seriously interfere with
> the education or training of the other
> children, those who are in moral danger,
> children guilty of repeated delinquency,
> those suffering from temperamental
> abnormalities - in a word children who are
> in need of care or control under the
> Mental Deficiency Acts and cannot receive
> the care they require except in certified
> institutions. (Report of the Mental
> Deficiency Committee: 1929, Part I,
> para.131)

The Committee was also concerned with the proper classification of mental defectives in institutions:

> The modern institution is generally a
> large one, preferably built on the
> Colony plan, taking defectives of all
> grades of defect and all ages. All, of
> course, are properly classified according
> to their mental capacity and age.
> (Report of the Mental Deficiency
> Committee: 1929, Part III, para.19)

The concern with proper classification led the Committee to stipulate a minimum size for each institution so that there would be adequate space for a proper classification of patients:

> The size of the central colony is
> important. It should make separate
> provision for both sexes of all ages and
> all grades, with separate detached villas
> for each class. The minimum number of

groups for which it is found in practice
that provision should be made is ten, six
of adults and four of children, and if
each adult group consists of 50 patients-
and a smaller number is uneconomical -
and each children's group of 40, it will
be seen that the smallest colony that
can provide proper classification must
probably take 460 patients. (Report of
the Mental Deficiency Committee: 1929,
Part III, para.71)

The 1931 Departmental Committee on the
Construction of Colonies also exhibited a concern
with "proper classification" of patients. It made
proper classification a major concern:

All our witnesses agreed on one point
and that was the need, even in the
smallest colony, for proper classification
of the patients. Many matters affect the
success and smooth working or otherwise
of a colony, but none is of such
importance as this matter of grading the
patients into appropriate groups, and
accommodating them in villas constructed
to meet the needs of each special class.
(Report of the Departmental Committee on
the Construction of Colonies: 1931,
para.15)

Like the Mental Deficiency Committee, the
1931 Departmental Committee felt there was an
irreducible minimum size for classification, which
it felt was 500 patients otherwise:

Epileptics, whether mild or severe,
troublesome patients and immoral and
criminal patients would be mixed with
quiet, harmless and so far innocent
good workers to the great detriment of
the latter.(Report of the Departmental
Committee on the Construction of Colonies:
1931, para.17)

Special Routine
The concept of the colony was closely
associated with the organisation of inmates'
activities. The 1904 Royal Commission was
impressed with the ways in which American colonies

21

used patient labour as a means of reducing running costs. In Amercian colonies:

> Space and opportunity have to be provided
> for manual labour of all kinds. The
> institution develops into the "colony"
> ... and this becomes the centre of a
> large estate, with the object both of
> employing the patients and of furnishing
> as large a part as possible of the
> necessaries of the establishment by their
> labour. (Report of the Royal Commission on
> the Care and Control of the Feeble-Minded:
> 1908, para. 855)

The Commission commended the use of patient labour as a therapeutic measure. They discussed the organisation of patient activities at the State Custodial Asylum at Rome, New York State, in the following way:

> Dr. Bernstein discouraged any education
> in the ordinary sense of the word
> He stated it was useless in most
> cases, and, where it succeeded, did not
> make for happiness, but increased
> restlessness, and a desire to leave the
> institution. He would like the whole of
> the time devoted to manual work ... More
> than 50 per cent. of the inmates were
> actually occupied in cleaning floors
> or in domestic work of some trifling
> description ... Apart from domestic
> work, painting, repairing etc., the farm
> was the chief source of employment.
> (Report of the Royal Commission on the
> Care and Control of the Feeble-Minded:
> 1908, para.857)

The Mental Deficiency Committee had a similar attitude to patients' activities. They argued that all the activities of mentally defective children could be exploited for therapeutic purposes. For example they argued that institutional care was superior to ordinary school for defective children because in the institution there was no division between the activities of daily living and the children's training:

> the term "training" is here used in the

22

> widest possible sense, including even
> learning to walk, training in clean
> habits and in dressing. There is one
> great and important advantage which the
> child in an institution ... has over the
> similar type of child attending a Day
> School; he is being trained seven days
> a week and all day long, and what he
> learns out of school hours is often
> more important than what he learns in
> school. (Report of the Mental Deficiency
> Committee: 1929, Part II, para.68)

For the Committee, not only did each class of
inmate have its own physical location in the
institution, it also had its own special set of
activities:

> In the all-grade institution ... the high
> grade patients are the skilled workmen
> of the colony ... the medium grade are the
> labourers ... the best of the lower grade
> patients fetch and carry ... and quite the
> lowest grade are the drones for whom all
> the others work. (Report of the Mental
> Deficiency Committee: 1929, Part III,
> para.19)

Comment

The mental deficiency colonies reproduced
many of the features of 19th Century asylums.
Their establishment was justified in a similar
way. "Reformers", who advocated the establishment
of the colonies, argued that workhouses and other
institutions were not designed for mental
defectives and therefore could not ensure their
proper classification or control. They argued
that mental defectives formed such a distinctive
group with such special needs that they needed
their own special institutions. These
institutions would ensure proper classifications
by segregating mental defectives from the rest of
society and they would ensure that the activities
of mental defectives were efficiently and
effectively managed.

1.5 ANTI-INSTITUTION

Institutions continued to expand and enjoy
government support in England for about 150 years.

In the 1950's and 1960's the traditional large
scale institution came under attack. Initially
the attack came from academics and researchers
such as Goffman (1968), Townsend (1962), Morris
(1969) (for a more detailed discussion see Jones
and Fowles: 1984, Part 1, The Springs of Protest),
but increasingly the criticisms were accepted by
policy-makers and were cited as accepted facts in
official reports.

The criticisms of institutions were not new.
As Rothman has shown there were considerable
criticisms of institutions in the U.S.A. at the
beginning of the 20th Century (Rothman: 1980). In
England, Lomax published his acoount of his
experiences as an asylum doctor (1921, see Towers:
1984). The difference lay in the official response
to these criticisms. As Rothman argued "in the
years 1900 - 1940, neither the insane nor their
doctors returned to the community ... The asylum
never lost its centrality and its needs shaped the
outcome of all reform ventures" (Rothman: 1980,
pp.324-5). Since the 1960's there have been
serious official attempts to run down and even
shut institutions and to develop alternatives.
Institutions still retain a dominant position in
the residential care of dependants but the outline
of an alternative can be seen in various official
reports and in some small experimental units.
These statements and units consciously and
explicitly reject the institutional tradition and
in this rejection provide more information about
the distinctive features of institutions.

Normalization is one expression of this
anti-institutional ideology that has become
associated with the residential care of mentally
handicapped people. Advocates of the normalization
principle claim that it is now "an internationally
influential service paradigm" (Flynn and Nitsch:
1980, p.3). As an ideology it has had considerable
impact but it has not yet succeeded in displacing
institutions from their dominance of residential
services:

> Perhaps the greatest challenge currently
> facing normalization is the "theory-
> practice gap". This principle has
> met with widespread intellectual,
> judical, and legislative approval, on
> the one hand. On the other,
> implementation has frequently been

> sporadic and superficial, and, indeed,
> in many jurisdictions it can be said
> to have scarcely begun. (Flynn and
> Nitsch: 1980, p.3)

In the U.S.A. the concept has been developed by Wolfensberger and is associated with the work of the Eastern Nebraska Community Office of Retardation (Thomas, Firth and Kendall: 1978). Wolfensberger argued that a society could manage its deviant members in four ways, through the "destruction of deviant individuals, their segregation, reversal of their condition or prevention thereof" (Wolfensberger: 1974, p.24). He argued that the first two approaches should be unacceptable in our society and therefore the treatment of dependent people such as mentally handicapped people should be based on the prevention or reversal of their deviance. This forms the basis of normalization.

In England the concepts of normalization were publicised through the work of the Campaign for Mentally Handicapped People. Normalization has been used to criticise the consequences of institutional provision.

> A cause and consequence (of segregated
> services) has been the stigma attached
> to the mentally handicapped and the
> separate institutions for them.
> (Kendall and Moss: 1972, p.7)

Instead of being separated in institutions, mentally handicapped people should be integrated in community facilities:

> For the handicapped child, integration
> offers the opportunity to gain
> self-confidence and social skills to
> deal with the outside world and non-
> handicapped people ... Integration
> should offer a more normal environment and
> more relevant and wider social
> experiences... It should also enable the
> mentally handicapped to feel part of, and
> be part of their local neighbourhood.
> (Kendall and Moss: 1972, p.8)

Integration means that as far as possible mentally handicapped people should live at home and use the same facilities as other citizens. When they cannot and require residential care the challenge for normalization is to design facilities that are not institutions. The Jay Committee on Mental Handicap Nursing and Care provided one model for alternative residential facilities. Experimental units, such as the Dr. Barnardo's Intensive Support Unit for Profoundly Mentally Handicapped Children have operationalised this model. In the remainder of this section I shall examine this new model. I shall focus on the information this model provides about the general nature of the institutions.

The Use of Ordinary Housing

The Jay Committee was critical of all purpose-built residential facilities and felt that there was a tendency for all purpose-built facilities to be institutional:

> We are beginning to realise the influence of architecture on the nature of the social environment and we need to investigate whether the style of the new purpose built homes for mentally handicapped people is in fact perpetuating the old "institutional" approach to care. (Committee of Enquiry into Mental Handicap Nursing and Care: 1979, para.114)

Similarly the Committee argued that:

> A purpose built unit on the outskirts of a housing development or a town is not in our view "in the community". (Committee of Enquiry into Mental Handicap Nursing and Care: 1979, para.135)

To ensure that mentally handicapped people have a right to enjoy normal patterns of life in the community, the Jay Committee recommended that all residential facilities for mentally handicapped people should be provided in "ordinary houses, suitably adapted for those with additional physical handicaps" (para.135). The preference of the Committee was "for such homes to be in specially adapted private houses" (para.114). Although the committee accepted the need for more specialised regional or sub-regional

26

accommodation, it felt that "wherever possible
these homes should share as many of the
characteristics of normal living which we envisage
in our staffed local homes as possible"
(para.147).

The Jay model of care has been
operationalised in Dr. Barnardo's Intensive
Support Unit in Liverpool. The I.S.U. is one of
several experimental schemes funded by the
D.H.S.S. to move all mentally handicapped children
out of long stay hospitals. The Secretary of
State for Social Services has accepted that large
mental handicap hospitals are no place for
children to grow up in. The number of children in
these hospitals has fallen rapidly from 7,100 in
1969, to 3,900 in 1977, to about 2,000 (D.H.S.S.:
1971, D.H.S.S.: 1980, D.H.S.S.: 1981). However the
remaining children are more difficult to place in
alternative care in the community as most need
special faciities because of their profound
handicap or behaviour problems. The Intensive
Support Unit is for profoundly mentally
handicapped children. The Unit admitted its first
children in July 1983 and was formally opened by
the Secretary of State for Social Services in
December 1983 (Ong and Alaszewski: 1984).

A major distinguishing feature of the
Barnardo's scheme is the use of ordinary housing.
The Unit has been established in 4 bungalows, each
with places for 2 children, in a newly built
middle class housing estate in Liverpool.
Alterations to the bungalows have been kept to a
minimum. Externally there are no signs that the
bungalows are any different to the other houses on
the estate. In one of the pairs of bungalows, the
builders altered the incline of the drive to make
it easier to push wheelchairs from the pavement to
the front door but a visitor would not notice this
alteration. Internally alterations have also been
kept to a minimum. The architect has widened some
of the corridors, installed special baths and
fitted boxed radiators. Apart from the bathroom,
a visitor would find the bungalows much the same
as other houses on the estate with the same
kitchens, fitted carpets and three piece suites in
the living rooms and ordinary beds in the
bedrooms.

In his speech at the formal opening of the
Unit, the Secretary of State emphasised the use of
ordinary housing:

> This is a unique and exciting new project.
> The houses here are not specially
> designed and built for mentally
> handicapped people. Apart from a few
> adaptations they are just the same as the
> houses in which their neighbours will be
> living. The houses are so normal and
> ordinary that anyone could be forgiven for
> not realising what an achievement they
> represent in providing for such severely
> mentally handicapped children.
> (D.H.S.S.: 1983)

An Emphasis on the Individual

Associated with the emphasis on ordinary
houses in the new ideology of residential care is
an emphasis on the individual care rather than the
care of groups or classes of inmates. The Jay
Committee repeatedly stressed the importance of
individuality and individual treatment. One of
their three broad sets of principles was that
"mentally handicapped people have a right to be
treated as individuals" (Committee of Enquiry into
Mental Handicap Nursing and Care: 1979, para.89).
Similarly in their description of the role of
residential staff they emphasised the importance
of individualised care:

> The staff must be able and encouraged to
> see each child as someone for whom their
> whole thrust of care is directed towards
> the development of all their capacities
> to the fullest potential. (para.118)

The Jay Committee believed there is a link
between smallness and individual treatment of
residents.

> whereas a 40 bed ward was regarded as
> small by comparison with a 70 bed ward
> 15 years ago, many people now think of
> "small" as meaning a maximum of 6 children
> in a house ... In this home (as envisaged
> by the committee) the small group of
> familiar people who care for him will
> provide opportunities for the child to
> develop emotionally ... socially and
> intellectually. (paras. 114 and 117)

The Jay Committee, after some disagreement,

agreed to avoid all categorisation and
classification of mentally handicapped people and
to concentrate instead on individuals and the
programmes they required:

> there was a group of Committee members who
> were highly reluctant to approach the task
> (of the committee) by attempting to
> categorise or identify "special groups"
> preferring to view each mentally
> handicapped person as having needs that
> might be special... On the other hand,
> there was another group of members who
> felt that we were neglecting or ignoring
> the needs of these "special groups"...In
> the end we had to set ourselves a number
> of ground-rules. The first was that we
> would try to avoid a "categorisation
> of special groups" approach. We
> preferred to consider each individual as
> having a unique constellation of general
> and special needs which were unlikely to
> be met by trying to match a particular
> group of residents to a particular kind
> of building. (paras. 98-99)

In the Dr. Barnardo's Unit the emphasis on
individual treatment permeates the organisation
and operation of the Unit and is referred to in
the unit as child centred care. Perhaps the most
distinctive feature of the individual care
approach is the use of link workers. The majority
of the care of the 8 children in the Unit is
provided by 10 residential social workers. 8 of
the 10 are titled link workers. Each link worker
is given prime responsibility for the care and
development of one of the children. Although the
link workers do not provide 24 hour care for their
child, they provide as much of their child's care
as possible and when they are on duty they are
usually caring for their own child. The link
workers are responsible for developing and
implementing individual goal plans for their
child. Each child has a goal plan that specifies
developmental objectives and outlines methods for
achieving these objectives. The link workers, in
consultation with psychologists, design the plans,
use the plans to coordinate the activities of all
individuals who come into contact and monitor the
progress of the children in relationship to the

plans. They are responsible for maintaining records of their child's activity and progress and for preparing information for 6-monthly reviews of the child.

Compared to traditional institutional methods of care in which groups of inmates are cared for by groups of staff, the link worker system is both expensive and inefficent. In the institutional system staff are interchangeable. In the link worker system they are not. The staff rotas have to be carefully designed to maximise the contact between the link worker and his or her child. There is only limited sharing of staffing resources between houses and unforeseen crises are more difficult to cope with. These costs are recognised in the Intensive Support Unit but it is felt that they are justified by the individual treatment of the children.

Normal Patterns of Living

Whereas the institution created its own distinctive pattern of activities, the advocates of the new style of residential facilities stress the importance of maintaining normal everyday rhythms of life in residential facilities.

The Jay Committee's first broad principle was that "mentally handicapped people have a right to enjoy normal patterns of life within the community" (Committee of Enquiry into Mental Handicap Nursing: 1979, para. 89a). It stated that "mentally handicapped people should be able to develop a daily routine like other people" (para. 91h). In its discussion of the organisation of the residential facilities the Committee stressed the importance of the normal experiences of every-day life:

> The small unit which we envisage is a place
> where residents and staff live together as
> a unit, a place where meals are cooked,
> washing-up is done and tradesmen are seen.
> In such small homes ... the child will
> experience as normal a life as possible...
> the contribution of those in the
> surrounding neighbourhood will be of high
> importance, and neighbours, shop-keepers
> and friends will play their part.
> We want the children to see the milkman
> and, however small they are, to be taken
> out shopping. This means that the social

> unit is one in which the staff are not
> enclosed but share many aspects of daily
> living with the children. (paras. 116
> and 119)

The Dr. Barnardo's Unit also places great
emphasis on creating and maintaining normal
patterns of life. This normal rhythm of life is a
central part of the definition of normalization
adopted in the Unit:

> normalization means making available to all
> mentally retarded people patterns of life
> and conditions of everyday living which
> are as close as possible to the regular
> circumstances and ways of life of this
> society. (Ong and Alaszewski: 1984, p.3)

During the course of our research in the
I.S.U., we conducted a study of the pattern of
life in the I.S.U. and we found it very different
to the pattern of life in the mental handicap
hospital.

> The I.S.U. was very different to the
> hospital. The children's daily lives and
> routines in the I.S.U. were not governed
> by a rigid routine of basic care
> activities. A daily routine could be
> identified and it was more marked during
> the week when the children had to be
> prepared for school but it was a fairly
> flexible routine, more like the routine in
> a normal household. The Residential Social
> Workers in the I.S.U. had to provide the
> children with the same basic care as the
> staff in the hospital, but were concerned
> to subordinate the performance of these
> activities to the provision of stimulation
> for the children. These basic care
> activities were performed in a different
> way. For example the R.S.W.s talked to
> the children while they were feeding them.
> The R.S.W.s did not see themselves as
> acting on the children, rather they tried
> to involve the children in these
> activities and to use activities such as
> bathing as a means of stimulation and
> play. Sometimes this meant that
> activities took longer than they did in

hospital but the R.S.W.s felt a need to
give the children more time.
At weekends the routine was difficult to
identify and the I.S.U. acquired a very
different character. The whole pace of
life was more leisurely and the level
of social interaction rose considerably
during the weekend. Staff arranged many
leisure activities for the children at
weekends and used these activities as a
means of stimulating the children.
The staff/child interaction in the Unit
was not restricted to the performance of
basic care activities. All the staff in
the Unit spent time interacting with the
children in a variety of ways. They
provided the children with therapy,
either through physiotherapy or through
goal-plans. They played with the
children and they cuddled and kissed the
children. The staff spent a lot of time
talking to the children and trying to
get responses out of them. (Alaszewski,
Eccles and Ong: 1984, p.61)

Comment
     The development of new types of residential
facilitities is a reaction to and a conscious
rejection of the traditions of the institutions.
Institutions were specially designed and purpose
built. The new residential facilities make use
of existing buildings, especially private houses.
Institutions created and maintained
classifications by segregating inmates from other
classes of people and by separating different
classes of inmates. The new units are so small
that no classification can develop, the residents
must be treated as individuals and they aim to
integrate residents into the community.
Institutions structure inmates' activities through
special routines. The new units aim to reproduce
the rhythms of normal domestic life.

1.6 CONCLUSION

     Institutions for dependants were a product of
reforms that took place at the beginning of the
19th Century. Reformers exposed conditions in
existing facilities and proposed radical reforms
with the establishment of new institutions. These

new institutions had different functions and served different categories of dependants but they shared characteristics. Unlike the madhouses and gaols they replaced, they were not housed in converted private houses but in specially designed buildings with distinctive architecture. These buildings separated the institution and its inmates from the rest of society. Internally the buildings created a structure of subunits that could be used for the proper classification of inmates. Associated with this spatial structure was a distinctive temporal structure of inmates' activities. All the activities of inmates were subject to scrutiny and control.

When new problem groups of dependants, such as mental defectives were identified, the institution provided a suitable model for their care and control. Mental Deficiency Colonies had their own distinctive characteristics but they exhibited the same underlying features as other institutions; special architecture, segregation, classification and special routines.

The concept of the institution is now under attack but the new normalised residential facilities emphasise the defining features of institutions by their conscious rejection of these features. These new residential facilities are negatives of the institution. Institutions were established in specially designed and built facilities. The new facilities use ordinary houses. Institutions segregated and classified large groups of dependants. The new facilities seek to integrate individuals and to reduce their dependency. Institutions structured inmate activities into special institutional regimes. The new facilities seek to establish and maintain normal everyday activities.

I can now extend the definition of institutions I provided at the start of this chapter. Not only are institutions organisations in which inmates are dependent on staff for some or all of the basic necessities of life but they are also large organisations with distinctive buildings that separate inmates from the rest of society, that classify inmates into groups and that structure their everyday activities through an institutional regime. Although there is nothing new about this extended definition, it does highlight the distinguishing characteristics of institutions. Since institutions have persisted for so long, the classification of inmates and the special routine must have a distinctive meaning and function. From historical sources it is difficult to identify this meaning and function. The only way this can be done is through the detailed case study of one functioning institution. The rest of this book is devoted to identifying the meaning and function of the classification of patients and the structure of the activities in one mental handicap hospital.

CHAPTER 2
THE JANE EAGLE HOSPITAL STUDY

2.1 INTRODUCTION

In this chapter I describe my research in one mental handicap hospital. The chapter is divided into three sections. In the first, I describe why I did the research and how my ideas developed during the different phases of my contact with the hospital. In the second section, I describe the theoretical background to my research methodology. In the third section, I discuss the methods I used in my study. The lay reader should find the first section relatively easy to follow. However the second and third sections are rather more difficult to read and unless you are particularly interested in social science research methodology I advise you to miss them.

2.2 A NATURAL HISTORY OF THE JANE EAGLE STUDY

In this section I shall provide a short account of how the project on which this book is based, developed. The discussion here is intended to supplement the methodological analysis in the rest of the chapter. In the rest of the chapter I focus on one part of the project only, the field work phase. However as all projects undergo evolution, this preface is intended to put that discussion in context. I have modelled this biographical and intellectual account of the development of my project on Whyte's methodological appendix to his study of Street Corner Society (Whyte: 1955, "On the Evolution of Street Corner Society").

Whyte's account highlighted the evolution of his study from a vague interest in slum life to an intensive participant observation study of one slum. Not only did the data for research emerge from the field work but so also did the analytic framework in which these data were collected. Furthermore, since Whyte used participant observation techniques rather than survey methods, the development of his project was linked with his own personal involvement in the field work. Whyte's approach created special problems of evidence. It is very hard to check on the validity of the data presented in his final report. The reader must largely either accept or reject the evidence presented. There is little the reader can do to test it or to judge how fairly it is reported. Whyte's response to this problem was to give a detailed account of the development of his study.

Becker has attempted to formalise this approach in a "natural history of research" (Becker: 1958). This approach would involve

> presenting the evidence as it came to the
> attention of the observer during the
> successive stages of his conceptualisation
> of the problem. (Becker: 1958, p.660)

In this section I shall give a biographical account of the evolution of my project and show how the different stages of development were associated with different problems.

Stage 1. Naive Participation
Like many postgraduate projects, the origins of my project were fortuitous and can be traced back to experiences as an undergraduate (Newby traces his interest in deferential workers back to his undergraduate dissertation, Newby: 1977). My undergraduate course in social anthropology was interrupted by an illness. Being recently married and without any money, I needed a job. A newspaper carried an advertisement for jobs in a mental handicap hospital. No training or qualifications were needed, the pay was reasonable and couples were encouraged to apply.

My first contacts with the hospital created a set of problems. These problems remained an important driving force behind the project and one of the objectives of my study was to resolve them. Loosely these problems can be labelled anthropological as they were a product of cultural

conflict. The culture of the hospital was so
different from any I had previously experienced
that there was much I could not understand and
many actions and statements I found strange,
distasteful, even shocking. Since the initial set
of problems created by first contact remained
important in the project I shall discuss my
initial impressions in detail. (I did not keep
any record of this interview and my account is
based on my recollection some 2 years later.)

Before I applied for the job, I went with my
wife to the hospital for an interview. As we had
little knowledge of and could not differentiate
between, mental illness and mental handicap, we
went initially to the local psychiatric hospital.
When we finally found the mental subnormality
hospital we were interviewed by the Senior Nursing
Officer. He stressed the unpleasant aspects of
the job. For example he asked if we would be able
to change incontinent patients or wash fully grown
men? However I found the SNO's implicit pessimism
more disturbing. I remember asking if patients
ever left the hospital and being shocked by the
negative answer. I subsequently discovered that
the SNO had been exaggerating but he was
articulating the general pessimism of the staff. I
was and still remain concerned about this
pessimism.

Despite the SNO's shock tactics, we decided
to apply for the jobs at the Jane Eagle Hospital.
I was allocated to Kestrel Ward and my wife to
Ravensbourn Ward. We arrived late for the first
shift and I had difficulty in getting into the
ward. All the doors were locked and I had not
been issued with any keys. When I did eventually
get in, the charge nurse told me to go into the
dayroom and observe the patients. I had no idea
what I was meant to do but he unlocked the dayroom
door and I went in. I was absolutely terrified by
what I met. There were 20 fully grown men and 10
or so large boys - some milling around, others
sitting in chairs. There seemed absolutely no
order in their movements and my overwhelming
impression was one of disorganisation and chaos.
Nothing in my previous experience had prepared me
for a situation like this. I felt both confused
and frightened.

After the shock of the first day I began to
see the order and organisation behind the chaos.
Although the behaviour of different patients on

the ward was idiosyncratic, it was also very predictable. One patient would sit in a chair and masturbate all day. Another would spend all day walking round the chairs. Yet another would run about flicking his hands. My socialisation had begun. Ward staff showed me how to understand the patients. They could, on this ward, be roughly divided into three categories:

1. the "duds" who were very dependent. They were doubly incontinent and had to be fed a soft diet. The "duds" were defenceless and were often the victims when other patients were upset;

2. the "disturbed patients", who were relatively independent. They were continent and could feed themselves. These patients were subject to swings of mood and when upset would "take it out" on the "duds";

3. the rest, who were the majority. Most could feed themselves and were generally continent but there was the odd accident of bowel and bladder control. They had moods but when upset they did not (usually) attack other patients.

These categories made life on the ward predictable, indeed after a while boring. Most shifts were easy. The duds had to be fed and changed but the rest were little trouble or work. The odd shift, when one of the disturbed patients was "up the stick" was more exciting. I learnt to enjoy these shifts because it was possible to display fast reactions and skill thereby preventing anyone getting hurt and "bringing down" the disturbed patient.

The relationship between staff and patients was physical and often rough. It was not unusual for patients to be slapped and it was easy to accept this physical relationship. Although I would not now condone this behaviour, although at the time my own behaviour was not significantly different from that of other nurses, I would differentiate it from brutality - a systematic physical assault on a patient. I only witnessed two such incidents. This type of incident raised important problems in the ethics of field work. In the first incident I intervened because I was employed on the ward and my primary responsibility was to the patients. In the second I did not. It

occurred during the field work phase of my
project. I put my field work before patient care.

My wife worked on Ravensbourn Ward and
occasionally I worked overtime on the ward. The
work on Ravensbourn was very different to that on
Kestrel. The patients were very dependent, few
could walk or feed themselves and everything had
to be done for them. There was more physical work
on Ravensbourn. Most of the patients had to be
fed, washed and changed and this involved a lot of
lifting and carrying. There were no disturbed
patients, so there were fewer problems of
control.

Occasionally I worked a shift on Magpie Ward.
This ward was different from both Ravensbourn and
Kestrel. Most of the patients were fairly
competent. They could wash and even bath
themselves. They could lay the tables and help
serve out the meals. They could even talk to
you. The work was not as heavy or as physical as
the work on Ravensbourn and was more interesting
than the work on Kestrel.

In the terminology of the nurses at the
hospital, Kestrel was a low grade ward, Magpie a
high grade ward and Ravensbourn a cot and chair
ward. Although individual nurses had different
preferences for the type of ward they liked to
work on, most preferred high grade wards. This was
a source of tension amongst nurses since the high
grade wards had the lowest establishment of
nurses. Although the wards were also divided into
adult and child, male and female, the tripartite
division into low grade, high grade and cot and
chair seemed the most important division between
wards. This division was related to the type of
work on the ward, the general atmosphere on the
ward and the attitude of staff.

By the time I returned to my studies, I had
become a fully socialised member of the culture. I
lived in a hospital house, participated in the
social life of the hospital and generally accepted
the actions and beliefs of the staff. Indeed my
own actions and attitudes to the patients were
similar. I was puzzled by the difference between
life in the hospital and life outside. It seemed
that the hospital had its own life divorced from
the world outside. When I entered the hospital,
or more especially the ward, I became involved in
a special set of relations or preoccupations -
would John be "up the shoot" today? Would Belinda

take forty minutes to feed? Would Tony run off
again? Thus Stage One ended with my acceptance of
the hospital culture but also with an awareness
that it was very interesting and different, i.e. a
suitable subject for a study.

Stage Two : Preparation.
My socialisation into the hospital culture
provided me with a ready made research topic. I
was interested in social anthroplogy and wanted to
do field work but did not want to leave England.
Doing field work at the Jane Eagle seemed an ideal
compromise. The hospital seemed to form a
distinctive community with its own culture. In
some respects it was similar to the communities
traditionally studied by social anthropologists. I
had already established close relations with the
members of the community I wanted to study.
Since I was closely involved in the hospital,
I withdrew from the hospital and concentrated on
background reading. A survey of the literature
added a new problem to my original anthropological
problem. I realised that many of the attitudes
and much of the behaviour that I had come to
accept were subjects of considerable critical
comment. However most writers were not interested
in understanding these attitudes and behaviour but
were more interested in evaluating and changing
them. I was determined not to abandon my concern
with understanding but was prepared to accept the
case for change. Thus to the anthropological
problem was added the social policy problem.
The addition of a new set of problems created
difficulties in project design. From an early
stage I had thought of the project as an intensive
field study of one community. I wanted to see the
interrelations of different aspects of the
culture. However the predominant design of social
policy research was comparative. Limited aspects
of different institutions were compared and
evaluated. I was urged by my supervisor and others
to undertake a comparative study. My supervisor
summarised the reasons in the following way:

> I remain unconvinced of the viability of
> a "community" study of a single
> institution within contemporary society,
> since this assumes an autonomy and
> separation of the institution from the
> wider society which I do not feel is

> justified... I still feel the
> introduction of something of a comparative
> perspective either between institutions or
> between certain sectors of the hospital is
> desirable.

Although I accepted the force of this
argument, I still felt that much social policy
research was premature. It investigated only
limited aspects of the institutions and did not,
in my view, take sufficient account of the
actors' subjective frames of reference. It was
necessary to understand one culture properly
before comparing different cultures.

Thus the problems of understanding the
culture of the mental handicap hospital dominated
the development of my methodology. The work that
at first seemed to have most relevance to my
problem was Silverman's overview of organisational
theory (Silverman: 1970 and 1975). Silverman
argued that the dominant view of organisations
based on systems theory treated organisations as
if they were things. Instead, drawing on the work
of Weber, he emphasised the subjective
interpretation of the actors. The organisation
could be seen as groups of actors with their own
objectives and beliefs. This view of
organisations fitted well with my reading of
Belknap's study of a state mental hospital.
Belknap showed the relationship between a set of
ideas about the nature of the patient behaviour
and condition and the working of the hospital
(Belknap: 1956).

I chose to use these ideas as the framework
for my own study. I intended to study how the
hospital structure reflected ideas about the
patients. I expected that different participants,
e.g. relatives, senior staff, ward staff,
therapists, would hold different views. Therefore
I planned a preliminary series of semi-structured
interviews with the different participants to find
out how they saw the patients and how they viewed
the organisation and function of the hospital. I
submitted my preliminary plans for research to the
hospital authorities and received conditional
approval.

Stage Three : Collecting the Evidence
After I received the conditional approval of
the project from the hospital authorities, I

concentrated on developing schedules of questions
to be covered in the interviews. When I had
reached an advanced stage, I submitted the
interview schedules to the hospital authorities
for final approval. The results were unfortunate.
There was a long delay and then plans for
interviewing hospital staff were accepted but
those for interviewing relatives rejected.
Furthermore all contact with relatives was
forbidden. The consultants argued that the
relatives were psychologically vulnerable and that
all contact with parents must be limited to
qualified staff. This decision was a shock. I
had been working on the assumption that I could
examine the work of the hospital from a variety of
perspectives. Without the relatives' view this
was impossible. Since I was more than half way
through the three year project I had little time
to adjust to the situation. I could either examine
the relatives' perspective or that of the hospital
staff. Since all my investment of time so far had
been spent in the hospital, I chose to concentrate
on the hospital staff.

The need to limit research to the hospital
staff meant a shift in emphasis. Interviews with
relatives would have provided a range of views
about the nature and organisation of the hospital.
Unlike the staff they were not socialised into the
hospital culture and there was less pressure on
them to accept the dominant view. Limiting the
research to the staff meant an increased emphasis
on shared views that were common currency amongst
the staff.

As I had worked in the hospital, I already
had a feel for its culture. I was already aware
of many of the attitudes of the staff, especially
the nurses, and of many of the strategies that
they used to cope with everyday life in the
hospital. I needed ways of collecting systematic
evidence about these attitudes and strategies. I
divided my research strategy in two parts. (For a
fuller explanation of the rationale of my methods
see the rest of this chapter.) In the first part
I interviewed staff about the hospital. I used a
schedule of questions to generate talk about the
hospital and its patients. This elicited evidence
about the different ways in which staff classified
the patients, especially the importance of
grouping wards and patients into high grade, low
grade and cot and chair groups.

In the second part I adopted a more passive, less intrusive role. I also recorded talk but this time talk initiated by and structured by staff. The regular case conferences and staff changeover periods were good opportunities for listening to and recording staff talking about their current preoccupations. Staff also recorded their current preoccupations in ward report books and patient records. Again these were useful sources. Finally on each type of ward I made structured records of staff-patient interactions.

Stage Four : Analysing the Evidence

Glaser and Strauss (1967) have distinguished two styles of research in the social sciences, hypothesis testing research and hypothesis creating research. They argue that these two styles of research follow different patterns of development. In hypothesis testing research, the researcher starts with clear hypotheses derived from existing theory, or uses well defined research procedures to gather data, usually quantitative data, in such a way as to test the hypotheses rigorously. Hypothesis testing research follows a three phase model of research common in the natural sciences. The boundaries between selection of hypotheses, collection of data and analysis of data are clearly drawn. In hypothesis generating research, there is no such neat, well defined model for research. The research worker simultaneously collects data, analyses them and creates hypotheses. Furthermore the researcher is more closely involved in the material. Whereas the hypothesis testing researcher can adopt a neutral role, arbitrating between hypothesis and evidence, the hypothesis creating researcher is more actively involved in selection and interpretation.

My research fitted neither of Glaser and Strauss's categories. Essentially my research was interpretative. The objective was to understand the culture. These objectives were summarised by Geertz in the following way:

> Believing, with Max Weber, that man is an
> animal suspended in webs of significance
> he himself has spun, I take culture to
> be those webs, and the analysis of it to
> be therefore not an experimental science
> in search of law but an interpretative one

> in search of meaning. (Geertz: 1973, p.5)

This interpretative science shares many of the problems of hypothesis generating research - it is difficult to separate the research from the object of research. Moreover these problems are exacerbated by the special role of theory. It is not an end, it is a means to an end - an essential tool in the process of understanding.

> Although one starts any effort at thick description, beyond the obvious and superficial, from a state of general bewilderment as to what the devil is going on - trying to find one's feet - one does not start (or ought not) intellectually empty-handed ... In ethnography, the office of theory is to provide a vocabulary in which what symbolic action has to say about itself - that is, about the role of culture in human life - can be expressed. (Geertz: 1973, p.27)

An important starting point in my analysis was the concept of culture. Traditional definitions of culture stressed the concrete and visible aspects of culture - human behaviour. Nadel described the subject matter of social anthropology in the following way:

> The subject matter of our enquiry is <u>standardized behaviour patterns</u>; their integrated totality is <u>culture</u>. (emphasis in the original text.) (Nadel: 1951, p.29)

Although Nadel also stressed observable behaviour, ideas and language play an important part in his analysis (Nadel: 1951, p.83).

In more recent analyses the emphasis has shifted from the visible manifestations of culture, to the underlying idea systems. Indeed in some styles of analysis, e.g. ethnoscience, the whole emphasis is on the underlying idea structures, which are subject to formal analyses, and behaviour is treated as an epiphenomenon. However I prefer Geertz's position. Geertz tries to keep the analysis of symbolic forms closely

tied to concrete social events and occasions
(Geertz: 1973, p.30). He described his approach
in the following way:

> Behavior must be attended to, and with
> some exactness, because it is through
> the flow of behavior - or, more
> precisely, social action - that cultural
> forms find articulation. (Geertz: 1973,
> p.17)

Although coherence or internal consistency
per se cannot be a test of the validity of a
cultural description, the consistency between
observable actions and implicit ideas can act as a
test. An example of this type of unity is Mauss's
description of Eskimo culture,

> The Eskimo have two ways of grouping, and...
> in accordance with these two forms there
> are two corresponding systems of law,
> two moral codes, two kinds of domestic
> economy and two forms of religious
> life. In the dense concentrations
> of the winter, a genuine community
> of ideas and material interests is formed.
> Its strong moral, mental and religious
> unity contrasts sharply with the
> isolation, social fragmentation and
> dearth of moral and religous life that
> occurs when everyone has scattered
> during the summer. (Mauss: 1979a, p.76)

In the case of the Eskimo the sharp division
between Summer and Winter highlights the unity of
ideas and activities in each sphere. Mauss used
the term "social morphology" to describe this
unity.

However in other cultures without clear cut
seasonal rhythms there are fewer contrasts to make
the underlying unity in each seasonal sphere
visible. Indeed the beliefs may be so well
internalised that no one questions or discusses
them. They are treated by competent members of
the culture as self evident or common sense.
Douglas encountered this problem in her research
amongst the Lele.

> Gradually I was able to relate these ideas
> (about the pangolin and other animals)

> within a broad framework of assumptions
> about animals and humans. These
> assumptions are so fundamental to Lele
> thought that one could almost describe
> them as unformulated categories through
> which they unconsciously organize their
> experience. They could never emerge in
> reply to direct questions because it was
> impossible for Lele to suppose that the
> questioner might take his standpoint on
> another set of assumptions. (Douglas:
> 1975, p.28)

Douglas's investigation of the Lele taken for granted views was facilitated by thesimplicity of Lele views and by her foreignness. Views that Lele took for granted, Douglas found strange and in need of further investigation and explanation. However the culture I was investigating was essentially a sub-culture. It used the language of and many of the assumptions of the dominant culture. Furthermore prior to the research I had been a member of both the dominant culture and of the sub-culture. How could I make the taken for granted assumptions explicit.

Nadel's discussion of culture suggested a useful starting point. Nadel highlighted the centrality of language to social behaviour, "all social behaviour happens in a world of language, amidst and through verbal communication" (Nadel: 1951, p.38). Language both provides signals for social actions and is a framework used to organise the physical and social universe, i.e. a framework for action. Language organises the world by placing it into categories and classifying it.

Mauss in his analysis of the Eskimo stressed the importance of classification in the organisation of the Eskimo universe.

> The way in which both men and objects
> are classified bears the imprint of this
> fundamental opposition between the two
> seasons. Each season serves to define
> an entire class of beings and objects.
> ... One could say that the concept
> of summer and the concept of winter
> are like two poles around which
> revolves the system of Eskimo ideas.
> (Mauss: 1979a, p.76)

The Eskimo world view was implicit in the way they classified and divided their social and physical universe. Modern anthropologists have also been interested in classifications. Douglas summarised this interest in the following way:

> No doubt the first essential procedure for understanding one's environment is to introduce order into apparent chaos by classifying. (Douglas: 1975, p.32)

Thus a starting point in my analysis of the hospital as a sub-culture was an examination of the way in which the nurses organised their environment. Central to this environment were the patients, therefore a central theme of my research was staff classifications of the environment they worked in, the hospital.

2.3 GENERAL METHODOLOGICAL APPROACH

I defined the objective of my research as the study of the culture of a hospital for the mentally handicapped. I was interested in culture both as manifested in staff actions and in the ideas that lay behind these actions. I used different methods to investigate these two areas. In the remainder of this chapter I shall discuss the overall approach that guided my research.

The social researcher's choice of methods is related not only to the type of problem studied but also to his or her overall approach to social science research. Two broad schools of thought can be identified among research workers. There are researchers who believe that the social sciences have the same objectives and therefore should use the same methods as the natural sciences, and there are researchers who believe that the objectives of the social and the natural sciences are different and therefore the methods required in each area of study are different. The first perspective has variously been described as positivistic, scientistic and natural. Schroyer described this perspective in the following way:

> This positivist view holds: (1) that knowledge is inherently neutral; (2) that there is a unitary scientific method; (3) that the standard of certainty and exactness in the physical

> sciences is the only explanatory model
> for scientific knowledge... Knowledge
> is thus conceived as a neutral
> picturing of fact. This denies that there
> could be any predefinitions of knowledge
> by prior organization of our experience.
> (Schroyer: 1971)

It is hardly surprising that early social researchers tended to model their methods on those of the natural sciences. These methods were well established, were associated with high status academic activities and had produced good results in the natural sciences.

Schutz outlined some of the differences between social sciences and natural sciences by stressing the unique characteristics of the subject matter of the social sciences. He argued that the natural scientist could impose his own order on the material he studies by selecting which universe of nature and which facts and events therein were relevant to his purpose (Schutz: 1971, p.5). This order would have an explanatory value for the scientist but would mean nothing to the material ordered. In contrast the "order" created by the social scientist could mean something for the people studied. It was not only a basis for a dialogue with other scientists, it was potentially also the basis for a dialogue with the people studied. People could talk about their actions and what they meant to do and this information was important for understanding what they did.

Weber stressed the importance of the meanings that people attached to their actions.

> In "action" is included all human behaviour
> when and in so far as the acting
> individual attaches a subjective meaning
> to it. (Weber: 1947, p.88)

Animals and physical compounds cannot talk about their behaviour.

Although the ability to talk to the subject of research is a unique feature of social research, it creates its own problems. Social researchers must understand their subjects. Some social researchers talk unselfconsciously to their subjects and do not concern themselves much with the problems of understanding (Cohen and Taylor:

1977). However for others the problems of communication and understanding are a major issue. These researchers are concerned about understanding too much, not understanding enough or misunderstanding.

Understanding too much

Social researchers who are concerned about understanding too much, usually work in their own culture. They argue that to talk and understand each other, people must start from shared assumptions. These shared assumptions include not only the rules of language but also implicit agreements about the nature of the world. Therefore any act of communication contains not only overt messages but also covert implicit messages. Some researchers feel that the covert messages are more important than the overt messages and devote their attention to understanding the covert messages implicit in talking.

Schutz called these covert messages and implicit agreements common sense. Common sense knowledge was both a central interest and a central problem for Schutz. It was a central interest because the implicit agreements made social action and social interaction possible. It was a problem because the social scientist had to work within the framework of the shared assumptions and yet at the same time try to stand outside and understand them. Schutz described this problem in the following way.

> The thought objects constructed by the
> social scientists refer to and are founded
> upon the thought objects constructed by
> the common-sense thought of man living
> his everyday life among his fellow-men.
> Thus the constructs used by the social
> scientist are, so to speak, constructs of
> the second degree, namely constructs of
> the constructs made by the actors on the
> social scene, whose behavior the
> scientist observes and tries to explain
> in accordance with the procedural rules
> of his science. (Schutz: 1971, p.6)

Schutz's solution to the problem was complex. The scientist had first to adopt a special attitude of mind. He had to lose his personal

involvement in talk and social action and become a
disinterested observer.

> By resolving to adopt the disinterested
> attitude of a scientific observer - in
> our language, by establishing the life-
> plan for scientific work - the social
> scientist detaches himself from his
> biographical situation within the social
> world. (Schutz: 1971, p.37)

Having   detached   himself   from   his
"biographical situation", the scientist had to
then observe actions and create models of these
actions. He   created ideal worlds   in which
"puppets" were given typical motive patterns and
this produced the requisite action patterns. The
second stage was to check whether the typical
motive patterns   as postulated in   the model
conformed to those of common sense knowledge
(Schutz: 1971, p.37).
Hindess described Schutz's social scientist
as a "puppet master" and characterised his work in
the following way:

> The social scientist and historian flit
> around applying the categories provided
> by the nice philosopher to their
> plasticene figures until they are able
> to reproduce the behaviour observed in the
> situations they happen to be interested
> in.
> Their stories are constructed in such a
> way that each act "would be understandable
> to the actor himself as well as to his
> fellow men in terms of common-sense inter-
> pretation of everyday life." (Schutz:
> 1971, p.64)
> The story-teller, in other words, must use
> categories and situations that are
> already familiar to his audience. His
> stories must appear plausible. (Hindess:
> 1977, pp.76-77)

Although Schutz sketched in a general method
of understanding the concealed basis of human
actions, he did not develop it. Attempts have
been made to apply Schutz's approach to empirical
research. Cicourel, like Schutz, was interested
in those aspects of interactions that people take

The Study

for granted and was concerned about understanding
too much and taking too much for granted.

> Measurement in sociology - or more
> appropriately, observation, classification
> and labelling - is rooted in the "common
> body of understanding" and "common
> understanding of the language" in every-
> day life. Thus sociologists must operate
> "from inside" the society, using its
> native language (syntax and vocabulary)
> and its many undefined cultural meanings.
> (Cicourel: 1964, p.24)

Cicourel was also concerned with making
explicit the assumptions built into everyday talk.
In the following extract he referred to these
assumptions as "background expectancies".

> The sociologist must come to grips with the
> problem of making the background
> expectancies visible to the reader when
> describing or reporting the results of
> his investigations if the shortcomings of
> sociological research are to be overcome.
> (Cicourel: 1976, p.15)

Cicourel concentrated on the process by which
diverse social reality is transformed through
background expectancies into limited and
predefined categories. Cicourel argued that the
researcher must not only provide evidence of the
transformation but also the background
expectancies used to achieve the transformation.
However Cicourel was not very explicit about how
he isolated these background expectancies.

> The conversational and written materials
> must be used to show how particular
> interpretations were intended by the
> speaker or writer, forcing the researcher
> to relate the narrow or broad limits to
> alternative interpretations permissible,
> given a specifiable contextual setting.
> By continual reference to the materials
> themselves (and the unstated, as well as
> the seen but unnoticed background
> expectancies imputed to members and
> assumed by the observer), the researcher
> specifies how the actors subscribe to

> interpretations typical of the
> categories employed and thereby achieve
> rational (for the actor) decisions.
> (Cicourel: 1976, p.16)

In the end we only have Cicourel's version of
the background expectancies. He could present no
concrete evidence because actors were unaware of
their background expectancies. Hindess suggested
Cicourel's background expectancies were just one
observer's interpretation amongst many. He
described Cicourel's approach in the following
way:

> In his later work what is "out there" for
> any given individual appears as the effect
> of the work of his background
> expectancies in transforming his
> environment of objects into intelligible
> phenomena. The sociologist in his
> examination of the "knowledge" of this
> individual is enjoined to make visible
> the "unstated and seen but unnoticed
> background expectancies" together with
> the environment of objects which they
> transform. This position necessarily
> induces an inescapable circularity in
> which the prescibed comparison of
> observer's report and environment of
> objects is invariably displaced into the
> comparison of one observer's report with
> another's. (Hindess: 1973, p.23)

Not understanding enough

Social researchers working in other cultures
tend to suffer from the opposite problem. They
feel they do not understand enough. There are two
related problems: 1. the strangeness of native
thought and the difficulty of understanding it in
its own terms and; 2. the difficulty of
translating this thought into the researcher's own
system of thought in such a way as to retain its
uniqueness and difference. These two problems are
of course interconnected. A translation that
makes sense cannot be taken as conclusive evidence
of a faithful representation of native ideas, but
one that does not make sense indicates either an
inadequate translation or an inadequate grasp of
the native system of thought.

> The most baffling translations of foreign
> ideas are the shortest ones, presented out
> of context, as parts away from wholes.
> The Bororo told von den Steinen in 1894
> that they were parrots (Levy-Bruhl, 1910).
> The Nuer say human twins are birds (Evans-
> Pritchard, 1956: pp.128-34). The Karam
> say that the cassowary is their sister's
> child (Bulmer, 1967). In certain
> specifiable contexts the animal or human
> member of the class could be substituted,
> the one for the other, without affecting
> the meaning. But in the short synonym
> the translation of the copula "is" has
> almost certainly been badly rendered.
> (Douglas: 1975, pp.278-9)

Regrettably anthropologists are often
reticent about their methods. The anthropologist
has to learn the native language, talk to natives,
and record conversations, activities and
associated interpretations. Then he or she has to
make sense out of the records and write up a field
report, an account in his or her own language of
the culture (or part of the culture) studied.
However until recently little attention has been
paid to the analysis of these activities. They
have tended to be seen as skills learnt through
apprenticeship and not codifiable. Although more
attention is currently being devoted to these
activities they may still be described in rather
obscure analogies.

> Doing ethnography is like trying to read
> (in the sense of "construct a reading
> of") a manuscript - foreign, faded, full
> of ellipses, incoherencies, suspicious
> emendations, and tendentious commentaries,
> but written not in conventionalised graphs
> of sound but in transient examples of
> shaped behavior. (Geertz: 1973, p.10)

Ethnography can also be seen as a jigsaw
puzzle made up of recorded statements and observed
actions. The ethnographer tries to get the bits
to fit together into one integrated whole, and
sometimes returns to the pieces to achieve a
better fit. For example Douglas returned to her
fieldnotes after 20 years to achieve this fit
(Douglas: 1975, p.206). Bourdieu used the analogy

of map making to describe traditional anthropology.

> It is significant that "culture" is
> sometimes described as a map; it is the
> analogy which occurs to an outsider who
> has to find his way around in a foreign
> landscape and who compensates for his
> lack of practical mastery, the prerogative
> of the native, by the use of a model of
> all possible routes. (emphasis in the
> original text) (Bourdieu: 1977, p.2)

Misunderstanding
   Bourdieu concentrated on the way in which
ethnographic research distorted the reality it was
trying to capture. Bourdieu characterised the
anthropologist as an observer from outside who
listened. He asked artificial questions which the
natives answered in an artificial manner. Bourdieu
suggested that this artificial talk created three
types of distortion.

> In so far as it (the artificial talk
> between ethnographer and native) is a
> discourse of familiarity, it leaves
> unsaid all that goes without saying ....
> In so far as it is an outsider-oriented
> discourse it tends to exclude all direct
> reference to particular cases ...
> Finally, the informant's discourse owes
> its best-hidden properties to the fact
> that it is the product of a semi-
> theoretical dispositon, inevitably
> induced by any learned question.
> (Emphasis in the original text)
> (Bourdieu: 1977, p.18)

   In other words the integrated structures that
anthropologists uncover can be a product of their
methods rather than of the social reality they
study.
   Bourdieu argued that anthropologists treated
ideological models which justified different
customs and practices as the rules that generated
these practices. Therefore they neglected the
strategies, distributions of power and status that
gave concrete form to different instances of a
practice. These different strategies could give
the same practices different meanings. Bourdieu

discussed in detail patrilateral parallel cousin marriage in which a man marries his father's brother's daughter in Kabylia in Algeria. Anthropologists had traditionally treated all such marriages as equivalent but Bourdieu showed that in practice the meaning of the marriage depended on its social context.

> Informants constantly remind us by their
> very incoherences and contradictions
> that marriage can never be fully
> defined in genealogical terms, and that
> it takes on different, even opposite
> meanings and functions, according to its
> determining conditions. They also remind
> us that parallel-cousin marriages can be
> the worst or best of marriages depending
> on whether it is seen as voluntary or
> forced, i.e. depending primarily in the
> relative positions of the families in
> the social structure. (Bourdieu: 1977,
> p.49)

Bourdieu is not alone in criticising the legalistic approach and the rather rigid view of rules and norms implicit in the work of early anthropologists. The difference between the ideal and actual has been discussed by Levi-Strauss as the difference between mechanical and statistical models. Levi-Strauss differentiated between the two models in terms of scale, mechanical models are small scale and based on the relations that ought to exist between actual individuals. Statistical models are large scale aggregations of actual practices. He used the laws of marriage as an example.

> In primitive societies these laws can
> be expressed in models calling for
> actual grouping of the individuals
> according to kin or clan; these are
> mechanical models. No such
> distribution exists in our own society,
> where types of marriage are determined
> by the size of the primary and
> secondary groups to which prospective
> mates belong, social fluidity, amount
> of information, and the like. A
> satisfactory (though yet untried) attempt
> to formulate the invariants of our

> marriage system would therefore have to
> determine average values- thresholds;
> it would be a statistical model.
> (Levi-Strauss: 1968, pp.283-284)

Firth's contrast between social structure and
social organisation also traded on the difference
between ideal and actual behaviour (Firth: 1961,
pp.35-36). Barth's transactional model is similar
to Bourdieu's practical strategies. Barth
similarly stressed individual choice. "The most
simple and general model available to us is one of
an aggregate of people exercising <u>choice</u> while
influenced by certain constraints and incentives"
(Barth: 1966, p.1).

Bourdieu used the concept of "habitus" to
replace that of laws. He defined "habitus" in the
following way.

> The structures constitutive of a particular
> type of environment (e.g. the material
> conditions of existence characteristics of
> a class condition) produce <u>habitus</u>,
> systems of durable, transposable
> <u>dispositions</u>, structured structures
> predisposed to function as structuring
> structures, that is, as principles of the
> generation and structuring of practices
> and representations which can be
> objectively "regulated" and "regular"
> without in any way being the product of
> obedience to rules, objectively adapted
> to their goals without presupposing a
> conscious aiming at ends or an express
> mastery of the operations necessary to
> attain them and, being all this,
> collectively orchestrated without
> being the product of the orchestrating
> action of a conductor. (emphasis in the
> original text) (Bourdieu: 1977, p.72)

Discussion

Compared to natural scientists, social
scientists have an added dimension to their
research. They can talk to those they observe.
However this unique feature of social science
research is not without its problems. Researchers
have been worried about understanding too much,
not enough or misunderstanding. Although it is
generally acknowledged to be a problem, there is

no agreement about how the researcher should deal with it. Each seeks his own solution. However the work of Bourdieu is useful in drawing attention to the difference between official accounts that justify practices and the actual strategies that create specific practices and is closest to the approach I adopted in my study.

In some respects Bourdieu's concern with "habitus", the engrained cultural dispositions, attitudes of mind, set of habits, and its relation to practice is similar to Schutz's common sense, everyday, taken for granted assumptions. Whereas Schutz constructs models based on different assumptions and contrasts them with actual behaviour, Bourdieu would place more emphasis on the need for participant observation and practical experience in other cultures as the only way to grasp and feel the "habitus" of people living in them.

2.4 MY RESEARCH METHODS

In my research I used two complementary sets of methods, the first to develop formal accounts of the hospital and its structure and the second to understand the relationship between these accounts and the structure of social action in the hospital.

Formal accounts of the hospital culture
In Jane Eagle hospital the primary concern of the staff was the care and control of the patients. To achieve this the staff needed ideas about the needs and nature of the patients. However these ideas were implicit. They were taken for granted and therefore only indirectly articulated when staff discussed patients. Therefore I had to make these ideas explicit. I did this by creating artificial talk about the patients. The procedure I followed for generating this artificial talk was loosely based on procedures developed by ethnoscientists.

In ethnoscience a major research technique is artificial talk or interview, in some cases modelled on formal linguistic eliciting techniques. The techniques used by ethnoscientists and componential analysts concentrate on a rigorous analysis of the internal relationship of different domains of native life such as kinship

The Study

terminology or disease. The researcher delimits a
part of the natives' social and physical universe
e.g. the body, cooking or disease, and gets the
native respondent to talk about it (Frake: 1961,
Metzger and Williams: 1963a, Metzger and Williams
1963b, Hammel: 1969). The techniques I used did
not achieve the same level of sophistication or
rigour as I was concerned with relationship
between ideas and actions rather than on the
internal coherence of ideas. Stark provides a
useful example of this approach (Stark: 1969).
Stark wanted to find out how a group of South
American Indians (Quechua) perceived their bodies.
She did this by examining the structure and
interrelationship of the words that these Indians
used to identify parts of their body. The first
step in the procedure was to obtain a list of
words for different body parts. She did this by
pointing to parts of her own body and asking a
native respondent to name it. The second step in
Stark's procedure was an examination of the
interrelationship between the various names for
the body. Respondents were given two names, A.
and B, and asked to organise them in the form A is
part of B. Stark argued that if one word was
classified as part of another, then it must
represent a narrower and more specific part of the
body. Repeating this procedure Stark produced a
hierarchy of levels of body parts and a lexical
"map" of Quechua body parts. At this stage, the
analyses of lexicon of body parts was purely
formal and many studies of native perception end
at this formal stage; however Stark developed her
analysis a stage further.
    Loosely, this third stage can be described as
an analysis of the "meaning" of the lexicon of
body parts. In one sense their "meaning" is their
reference to parts of the anatomy but the lexemes
or parts of them are also used in other lexical
domains. Thus Stark developed her analysis by
examining the relationship between different
lexical domains. She examined the different
meanings of the same lexeme (or symbol) in
different contexts and the metaphorical
interrelationships between the contexts. For
example she established that various parts of the
facial anatomy were systematically differentiated
by lexemes which can be translated by the words
"hollow" and "rounded". These concepts of
concavity and convexity were related to words in

the Quechua geographical domain. Since these
lexemes were part of complex lexemes (two or more
simple lexemes) in the body parts domain and
simple lexemes in the geographical domain, Stark
argued that their primary position was in the
geographical domain and they were being used
metaphorically in the body parts domain. There
was also evidence of the reverse associations.
Stark summarised the situation in the following
way:

> In either case it may be possible to assert
> that the Quechua speaker's conception of
> the body as convex-concave contrasts may
> be the result of his conception of
> geographical topology, where contrasts
> between convex and concave entities
> exist on a far grander scale than on
> the body. (Stark: 1969, p.9)

Stark utilised a three stage procedure. In
the first she defined her universe of discourse
and the words associated with it. In the second
she examined the interrelationships of the words
in this domain. In the third she examined the
meaning of these words by examining the
interrelationships between this domain and others
in which the same words appeared. Loosely the
interviews used in the project followed this
approach. The method used was neither as neat nor
as tightly structured because the vocabulary used
was less specific, less systematic and had more
alternative references.

The domain was defined as the hospital's
"patients". The first stage was to obtain
the list of words associated with the
classification of "patients". The second stage
was to examine the interrelationships of these
words and the third to explore their meaning.
Since my focus was the sub-culture of the
hospital, I was especially interested in words or
terms that were unique to this setting.

All three parts of the analysis were based on
the same research instrument, a semi-structured
interview. The domain was defined as hospital
"patients". Stark organised her methodology in
two stages, in the first stage she obtained the
names for body parts and in the second phase she
obtained the hierarchical organisation of these
parts. In my research the hierarchical

organisation was more evident. The hospital, itself, formed a hierarchy. At the most inclusive level was the hospital itself. This included the physical fabric, the staff and all the patients. The hospital was divided into wards and departments. Again the wards were discrete buildings but they were also units of patients and units of staff. Finally the patients on each ward could be divided into groups. Although there was no specific subward division of staff to match the sub-classification of patients it was possible to identify some physical sub-division of space on the wards. Thus the hierarchy was not only a taxonomic hierarchy in that one term (e.g. hospital) covered a number of discrete terminological divisions made at lower levels (e.g. wards) but was also an organisational hierarchy of staff and a spatial hierarchy of buildings.

I used these three levels, hospital, wards and subwards as the main structure of my questions. I organised the questions starting at the highest level and moving down the hierarchy. I sought comparisons between different groups of patients at each level in the hierarchy. Whereas Stark had been a foreigner amongst the Quechua, I was, in some respects, a "native". Therefore in the interviews I stressed that I was to be treated as a foreigner, as someone who knew nothing about the hospital. In practice this did not seem to create a serious problem.

Although the precise content of the questions varied according to the position within the hospital hierarchy of the respondent, the usual order was as follows:

Question 1. How would you describe the patients in this hospital to someone who knew very little about the hospital?

Question 2. Do you think there are different types of patient in this hospital? If so how would you describe them?

Question 3. How would you describe patients on this ward (i.e. on which the respondent was currently working) to someone who knew very little about the hospital?

Question 4. (I shall discuss this question later.)

Question 5. *(Answers to Questions 2 and 3

were usually in terms of wards, i.e.
there are Seagull patients and Pelican
patients. The relationship between these
types were explored.) How are the
patients on this ward different from those
on _____? (name of the
other wards specified. This question
repeated for each of the types
specified.)
Question 6. Do you think there are
different types of patients on this ward?
If so could you describe them?

From these questions the following types of
response were obtained:

Question 2. ... How would you categorise
them?
Answer The only categories I would use are
high dependency and low dependency. The
ones on here (on Seagull Ward) are low
dependency. The ones on Beaver, Kestrel
and Ravensbourn are high dependency.

This respondent answered Question 5 in the
following way:

It (Seagull) is a much higher grade ward,
much higher intelligence, they can do a
lot more things for themselves, but
you have more problems.

From these interviews I extracted certain key
words. I defined these as key words because they
recurred and were central to the classifications,
ambulant/non ambulant, adult/child, male/female,
high grade/low grade/cot and chair. Using these
contrasts it was possible to generate a structured
"lexicon" of the hospital wards. Other unofficial
and official accounts of mental handicap hospitals
were examined to see if they contained the same
terminology (See Chapter Three).
The first two stages of Stark's procedure
were concerned with the terminology and its
structure. In the third stage she started to
identify the meaning and function of the
classification. This was a major concern of my
research and involved the procedures discussed in
the next section. However in the interview two
questions were specifically concerned with the

function (Question 4 and 7). These were as
follows:

> Question 4. What are the special problems
> that patients on this ward present?
> Question 7. Which patients on this ward
> present the greatest problem and why is
> this?

These questions were intended to emphasise
the practical aspects of the classifications and
therefore one aspect of their function.

The number of staff I interviewed is recorded
in Table 2.1. Numbers were not important as I was
not involved in a statistical investigation. I
was interested in the different ways nurses and
other staff classified patients.

The first set of research techniques was
aimed at making explicit staff theories about the
nature of the patients. These theories were
related to staff classifications of the patients
and the meanings they attributed to these
classifications. The semi-structured interview was
a means of promoting talk about the patients and
obtaining the classifications and associated terms
and I use the material from these interviews as
the basis of the second part of this book.

In the next part of this section, I shall
discuss the methods used to obtain the information
used in the third part of this book. These
methods were concerned with examining staff
actions and with examining the relationship
between the classifications, staff ideas about the
patient and practice. While the emphasis in the
second part of the book is on the classification
as a symbolic system and its expressive
dimensions, in the third part of the book I
discuss what is done in practice.

Actions and Practice

The artificial talk I have just outlined was
researcher initiated and structured. Therefore
the accounts it produced of the hospital, patients
and staff-patient relations, were accounts of what
ought to happen, the rules that ought to guide
behaviour, rather than accounts of what did
happen. As Bourdieu points out this type of
artificial talk artificially structures thought:

> Quite apart from the form which the

The Study

Table 2.1 <u>Number and type of respondents in the interviews</u>

Overall Staff Category	Sub-Category	Number of interviews
Senior Hospital Personnel	Doctors	3
	General Administrators	2
	Nursing Administrators	4
		—
	Total	9
		—
Nurses	Nurse Tutors	1
	Qualified Nurses	16
	Nurses in Training	17
	Unqualified Nurses	7
	Nurse Therapists	2
		—
	Total	43
		—
Other Professional Staff	Therapists	7
	Other	1
		—
	Total	8
		—
Other Staff	Domestics	5
		—
	Total	5
		—
Total Respondents		65
		—

> questioning must take so as to elicit an
> ordered sequence of answers, everything
> about the inquiry relationship itself
> betrays the interrogator's "theoretical"
> (i.e. "non-practical") disposition and
> invites the interrogatee to adopt a
> quasi-theoretical attitude. (Bourdieu:
> 1977, p.106)

Therefore these accounts needed to be accompanied by descriptions of actions, so that the relationship between the two can be explored. Whereas the "semi-theoretical" accounts were obtained by artificial talk, the descriptions of practice had to come from natural talk and natural action, i.e. talk and actions initiated and structured by the subjects of the research.

The structured talk showed that the tripartite system of classification of the patients into "cot and chair", "low grade" and "high grade" was a key element in the structure of staff-patient relations. Therefore I chose one ward from each type (and a therapy unit that covered all three) as sites for observation. On each unit I was interested in the current preoccupations of the staff and their relationship with the patients, and I used a variety of techniques to examine these relations including participation at case conferences, listening to staff talk, analysis of records and observation.

Case Conference   On each ward there were case conferences. At each conference two patients selected by the ward staff, were discussed by a panel of staff. These conferences were especially useful because ward staff selected "problem" patients for discussion, and the discussions brought together staff from different disciplines, nurses, therapists, psychologists, social workers and doctors. Thus it gave an opportunity to listen to talk about patients, and to listen to practical solutions suggested for practical problems. I took notes during the conference and wrote these notes into a fuller account later, usually the same evening.

Listening to staff talk   On each ward in addition to interviewing staff I engaged in unstructured talk. This was unstructured in the sense that I did not initiate the topic for discussion nor did

64

I try to structure the talk. I talked with ward
staff about current problems. Generally I did not
record the talk at the time but recorded it in
field-note books afterwards. Usually I wrote my
reports the same day but if for some reason this
was not possible then I made short notes as an
aide memoire as soon as I could be sure of
reasonable privacy. Structured talk was tape
recorded. Like the case conferences, the
unstructured talk was generally about problem
patients. The participation was usually restricted
to nursing staff (see Table 2.2) but occasionally
I recorded talk between nursing staff and visitors
to the ward (doctors and therapists). I found
that the best opportunity for listening to the
staff talking was at shift changeovers when the
nurses finishing a shift told the new shift about
the problems and difficulties they had
encountered.

The patients' notes were private records,
open only to a limited group of individuals
including myself. At the time of my research,
consultants and senior staff were discussing
whether to give unqualified members of the nursing
and therapy staff access to patients' notes. They
eventually gave these categories of staff
conditional and limited access. The patients'
notes include both routine records and records of
specific incidents. In the case of problem
patients the patients' notes provided a
fascinating record of the incidents, staff
interpretations and proposed methods of dealing
with the problems.

<u>Observation</u> I made general observations lasting
over the field-study period and these were
recorded in my field-note books. In addition on
the three wards I made two special types of
semi-structured observation. One set of
observations was concerned with meal-times, the
other with activities that took place during one
day, a Sunday.

On the ward, the key activities were
associated with the basic care of patients,
activities associated with sleeping,
eating/drinking and the removal of bodily waste or
dirt. Of these activities the easiest to observe
were those associated with eating. They were
clearly defined, taking place within clear
temporal and spatial boundaries. On each ward I

65

Table 2.2 Analysis of records of staff-structured talk
(derived from field note books).

Overall Staff Category	Sub-Category	Number of separated recorded episodes	Number of different individuals involved
Senior Hospital Personnel	Doctors	13	5
	General Administrators	5	2
	Nursing Administrators	17	5
	Total	35	12
Nurses	Nurse Tutors	4	2
	Qualified Nurses	51	21
	Nurses in Training	30	17
	Unqualified Nurses	22	11
	Nurse Therapists	3	2
	Total	110	53
Other Professional Staff	Therapists	15	7
	Others	5	4
	Total	20	11
Other Staff	Domestics	8	8
	Total	8	8
Total		173	84

observed and recorded seven main meals.

The recording procedure was straightforward. A pad of paper was prepared with the names of all the patients and staff on each sheet. A single sheet was used to record the dominant activities and interactions in a specific period of time. The actual periods used varied according to the pace of activities from about five minutes per sheet to about ten minutes per sheet.

In the recording the emphasis was on the overall pattern of activities and interactions, not the minute details of behaviour. This was all that was feasible for one unaided observer to attempt, given the particular situation and aims of my observations. Even with video recording equipment it would have been difficult to develop a comprehensive analysis of the behaviour of nearly 35 individuals. The size of task can be gauged from the fact that one anthropologist observing his wife in the kitchen recorded 480 elementary units of behaviour in 20 minutes (Harris: 1964, pp.74-75). I paid special attention to the start of each activity, e.g. the time at which each patient sat down at the table was recorded. I considered these broad descriptive categories adequate because I was interested in the variation of activity patterns between wards rather than the behaviour of specific individuals. I was also able to record many of the interactions that accompanied these activities. Again the emphasis was on the general flow and direction of interactions but more detailed records were made of exchanges that I found interesting.

The second type of observation was based on the pattern of activities over time. Since my objective was to contrast the activities between units I used the recording procedure described above. The overall time unit selected was a whole day (from the time of the patients' getting up to the patients' going to sleep, or in staff terms 2 day shifts). A Sunday was selected because the patients were on the ward the whole day. Two problems were encountered: 1. the wards were large places and on ambulant wards it was sometimes difficult to keep track of all the patients and 2. at times one or more patients left the ward. Usually I remained on the ward but in one instance I went with nurses to collect a patient who had left without permission.

Summary
    Whereas the artificial talk and interview created accounts of the hospital, this less intrusive approach was designed to obtain information and descriptions of activities. This information came from recording talk on the wards, at panel assessment and during staff changeovers and extracts from the ward records. Descriptions of activities came from structured observation.

2.4 COMMENT

    Social researchers are in a privileged position. They can not only observe behaviour but they can also talk to those they observe about their behaviour. Some researchers have accepted this opportunity unselfconsciously. However other researchers have been concerned about understanding too much or not enough, and about misunderstanding. Although there is general awareness of the problems, there is no accepted strategy for overcoming them.
    I adopted a two phase research stragegy. In the first part, I promoted artificial talk to identify the implicit assumptions staff had about the patients, the nature of their work and the hospital. I initiated and structured this talk through a schedule of questions. This strategy generated accounts on the nature of the patients and therefore the type of work involved. In the second part I concentrated on how the hospital actually worked. I had to avoid imposing an artificial (research) structure on staff talk. To do this I observed and recorded talk and activities organised by staff such as ward case conferences, change-over periods, ward records and meal-times. I examined ward records. I observed staff-patient interactions.

CHAPTER 3
THE STRUCTURE OF THE CLASSIFICATION OF WARDS

3.1 INTRODUCTION

Since Durkheim and Mauss's seminal study of
primitive classification (Durkheim and Mauss:
1969), the study of systems of classification has
played an important and sometimes central part in
the study of other cultures. Levi-Strauss has
argued that:

> Classifying, as opposed to not classifying,
> has a value of its own, whatever form the
> classification may take. As a recent
> theorist of taxonomy writes: "Scientists
> do tolerate uncertainty and frustration,
> because they must. The one thing that
> they do not and must not tolerate is
> disorder... the most basic postulate of
> science is that nature itself is
> orderly... All theoretical science is
> ordering..." The thought we call
> primitive is founded on this demand for
> order. (Levi-Strauss: 1972, pp.9-10)

The first step in understanding a culture has
often been to understand how members of the
culture classify and organise their environment.
However studies of classifications, especially
folk classifications, in our own culture have been
relatively neglected. Douglas has suggested a
reason for this neglect. Whereas we find the
classifications used by other cultures strange and
therefore feel they must be wrong, we find our own
classifications familiar and therefore they are
right and they reflect objective reality:

> Like the tribal peoples, we have
> internalised the classifications of our
> social group; we see no other kinds of
> reality. (Douglas: 1975, p.219)

However like the people in other cultures, we use our classifications for practical purposes - to make sense, to create control and to allow us to act - therefore there is no reason why they should not be subject to the same type of analysis. There are, of course, differences between the social contexts of classification in industrial societies and simpler societies, especially the complex division of labour in Western society and the more sophisticated modes of communication. I shall discuss these differences in Chapter Five.

In this chapter I examine the ways in which nurses at the Jane Eagle hospital classified patients. I examine two types of classification - the classification of wards and the classification within wards. Since wards were physically distinct entities (single storey villas), their classification had a visible concrete expression. The classifications within wards also had visible expressions, e.g. the arrangements of beds in the dormitories, the layout of tables at mealtimes, but these arrangements were less permanent. Therefore the classifications within wards were more variable both over time and between nurses.

3.2 THE CLASSIFICATION OF WARDS

In this section I shall discuss two aspects of the nurses' classification of wards, the terminology used by nurses to classify patients and the structure of nurses' classification.

The terminology of the ward classification

I choose to start my account with a lengthy statement made by a member of staff who had extensive experience of work on both the wards and the therapy units. The statement, transcribed from the tape-recording of an interview, classified the wards into three groups and provided a discussion of each group. The interview was artificial talk which should have been structured by the interviewer, however in this case the respondent introduced his own structure by jumping straight into a discussion of

the different categories of patients and omitting
any discussion of their general characterisation.

> Question - How would you describe the
>   hospital to somebody who knew very little
>   about them?

> Answer - I could divide it into groups for
>   people that didn't know much about it.

> Question - How?

> Answer - I would go straight to the cot and
>   chair wards to remove that obstacle. Cot
>   and chair wards generally have a very low
>   ability patient who is multiply
>   handicapped. These are the areas in which
>   I would place the public at risk in its
>   reaction, its response on first seeing the
>   patient, in shying away from a deformed
>   and vegetating mass of humanity.

This nurse used the terms "cot and chair",
"low ability", "multiply handicapped", "deformed"
and "vegetating" in his discussion of the first
group. Cot and chair was used as a label for this
type of ward and its patients and the other terms
were used more descriptively. The second group of
patients was discussed in the following way:

> Answer - Then you go onto the bizarre cases
>   that you get in the low grade ambulant
>   wards, like Woodfinch, Pelican, and to a
>   certain extent Kestrel ... One of the
>   things that strikes you immediately is the
>   erratic, unnerving, ant-like movement of
>   the patients around the ward. They strike
>   me like the movement of the bleep on that
>   T.V. ping pong game ... going from wall
>   to wall, and whenever you go in you
>   immediately draw their attention and they
>   come to you ...

> Question - How far do you think animal
>   comparisons are current in the hospital
>
>   (i.e. among nurses) for this sort of
>   patient.

> Answer - (pause) I feel that there's a

dualistic approach. Although staff have a degree of familiarity with patients as people, as individuals, none the less there are certain activities that these handicapped children/adults take up that are always going to be regarded as animal: defecating; pissing; throwing down food at mealtimes; ripping clothes; rocking. Which is not so much animal as unnerving ... (there's) a gut response ... a definite drive to stamp out this animal behaviour which leads to a uniformity of response, which processes patients and this is where you run into the effacing of personality and the unacceptable face of the institution.

This group of wards (and patients) was labelled "low grade". The description of the patients centres on their behaviour, which was described in anti-social terms - "erratic", "unnerving", "ant-like movement" and "the movement of a bleep on a T.V. ping pong game". Whereas the behaviour of cot and chair patients was described as "vegetating" the respondent was prepared to accept a description of the behaviour of low grade patients as "animal". In his discussion, the respondent recognised that this type of classification emphasised the common features of patients and underplayed the individuality of patients. The respondent recognised a third and final group of wards and patients.

Question - What about the third type of patient?

Answer - The third type. Well let's say you've got a reasonably well adjusted patient, some of the Leopard boys, some of the Magpie boys and some of the Seagull ... women, who seem to have adopted (sic) the paternalism of the hospital.

Question - Accepted?

Answer - And the formal paternalism of a ward like Leopard and find that within this security they can relate to the staff as children to adults, and be rewarded and be congratulated and

somehow lead an unreal existence.
Anyway they seem to be gratified as
much as they are disappointed. They
have their private sorrows that you
can't get at for a long time because
they aren't monitored as individuals,
not sufficiently in any case. But I'd
say they were reasonably well adjusted.

He did not label this group in the same way
as he labelled "cot and chair" and "low grade"
wards. He used the ward names, Leopard, Magpie and
Seagull, as labels. The behaviour of these
patients was described in social terms, "well
adjusted" and they related "as children to
adults". This nurse stressed the individuality of
this group of patients.

In summary, this respondent divided and
grouped hospital wards and patients into three
classes and associated the following terms with
each class:

Cot and chair, low ability, multiply
handicapped, deformed and vegetating;

Low-grade, erratic, unnerving, ant-like
movement, the movement of a bleep on
a T.V. ping-pong game, animal;

Well-adjusted, children.

Other accounts of the hospital provided a
similar grouping of wards and patients. All
tended to exclude one ward, Hawk ward, and divided
the other wards into three groups, cot and chair,
low grade and high grade. The following
classification of wards was derived from a written
report made by one student nurse. The student had
been asked to show visitors round the hospital and
had written an aide memoire for this purpose. He
submitted this to the senior nursing officer. This
report therefore represented an "official" account
for each ward. Hawk Ward was omitted from his
list but the other wards were labelled in the
following way:

Ravensbourn and Beaver Wards are both termed
as cot and chair wards ...
Drake Ward ... is a low grade adolescent
male ward.

Leopard Ward ... is an adolescent boys'
  ward, which is higher grade than
  Drake ...
Magpie is another male ward. This is where
  the highest grade male patients
  reside ...
Kestrel is yet another male ward. It is
  occupied by low grade adult men ...
Woodfinch. All the patients on this ward
  are low grade children, mainly girls.
Pelican Ward ... low grade adult female
  patients.
Seagull ... high grade adult female ward.

In this account the wards were grouped into
three classes, cot and chair ward, low grade ward
and high (or higher/highest) grade. There were
other classifications that cut across the grade
classification, i.e.classification by sex and
classification by age, but this account placed
greatest emphasis on the grade classification.

Classification by grade was the dominant
mode of classification amongst the nurses. It
was even seen as a type of reality that has to be
concealed from outsiders such as the patients'
parents.

Question - How would you describe the
  patients to someone who knew very little
  about the hospital?

Answer - Well, there are high grade,
  low grade and cot and chair. You wouldn't
  say that to the patient's parents because
  if they happened to have the low grade.
  I would say that we have patients who
  could do most things for themselves
  like Seagull and Magpie, we have
  patients who can do things for themselves
  with a lot of help like Drake, and
  patients who can't do anything for
  themselves like Beaver and Ravensbourn -
  the spastic ones. You have to be careful
  what you say to the parents because they
  are quite sensitive.

Not all respondents gave a fully developed
account of the grade classification, some
concentrated on one grade, e.g. one group of
wards. The trichotomy of cot and chair, low grade

and high grade was occasionally divided into or replaced by various dichotomies. For example the nonambulant cot and chair patients could be contrasted with the ambulant low grade and high grade patients. In the following interview low dependency high grade patients are contrasted with high dependency cot and chair and Hawk patients.

> Question - Could you categorise the
>   patients?

> Answer - The only categories I would use
>   are the high dependency and low
>   dependency. The ones here (on Seagull
>   Ward) are low dependency. The ones on
>   Beaver, Hawk and Ravensbourn are high
>   dependency.

Comment At the Jane Eagle Hospital nurses used various ways of grouping and classifying wards. One particular form based on a grade classification had a prominent position in their accounts. In the second part of this section I shall examine official and unofficial accounts from other sources to see if this same type of classification exists in other hospitals for the mentally handicapped.

Accounts from other hospitals
    If the classification I have identified in the first part of this section is an important aspect of hospital culture, then it should be evident in other hospitals with a similar culture. This is indeed the case.
    The usage of the terms high grade and low grade has been widely reported in studies of English mental handicap hospitals. I refer to these reports as unofficial when they appear to be based on private talk with staff in the hospital and official when they are based on "public" statements by service administrators. It is sometimes difficult, from published accounts, to ascertain the source of the information and therefore the status of the account. For example Jones's study of services for the mentally handicapped in one Hospital Region was based on information collected by a team. It appears that the information was processed through three levels. Each member of the team visited the hospitals in one area and collected fieldnotes.

75

These then formed the basis of a series of working reports written by different team members. Jones used these as the basis of the final report. (Jones: 1975).

Tyne, in his study of Parker Village Hospital, reported that "in the hospital itself patients were commonly referred to as "subnormals" and the terms "high-grade" and "low-grade" were almost universal" (Tyne: 1974, p88). He gave the following examples:

> A low-grade can't help himself - The high
> grades, like Fred, can do things for
> himself but he still needs the security
> of a villa. A low-grade can't help
> himself. He does things without reason.
> He can't understand ...
> High-grades are like normal people, but
> the low-grade have almost no I.Q. at all.
> The high-grade - his thinking is more.
> But the low-grade, you have got to do
> everything for him. (Tyne: 1974, p.88)

M. Bury in his study of "Yellow Ward" also reported the use of the term "high grade".

> the initial impact (of Yellow Ward) in (sic)
> the outsider is overwhelming. A crowd
> of weird faces and bodies, together
> with a battery of noises and smells,
> greets the visitor. Nurses on Yellow Ward
> itself tell how they thought the prospect
> of changing from a "high-grade" ward to
> Yellow Ward a daunting one. (Bury: 1974,
> pp.249-250)

Tyne and Bury appear to be using "raw" data i.e. the unofficial accounts of nurses. In other ethnographic accounts although the raw data are recognisable, the researchers have imposed an interpretative framework on it. Jones in her study introduced the term "back ward". This term was derived from the American literature on psychiatric hospitals and was not one used in the English mental handicap hospital. The term "back ward" is derived from the back wards in large 19th century asylums. Most English mental handicap hospitals were built in one of two phases, the 1920's and 1930's and the 1960's. The earlier phase was dominated by two storey "Board of

Control" villas, the second phase by single storey villas. In both phases, the villas tended to be grouped round a central administrative block. Therefore there are usually no back wards in the sense of villas located behind the others. However, it is clear from Jones's account "back wards" were low grade wards.

> The adverse features of ward management
> which they ("back wards") exhibit may be
> found in greater or lesser degree in many
> other wards, and they may become more
> common - for as the "good", high-grade
> patients are discharged to community care,
> so the hospitals will increasingly have
> to focus on those perceived as "low-
> grade". (Jones: 1975, p.96)

In a search for a logical taxonomy Jones found that the "back wards" created special problems. Having recorded the term "child" for all the patients in the hospital and for patients on high grade ward, Jones also recorded the use of the term "animal" on low grade wards. She explained this apparent inconsistency in the following way:

> The model of the hospital wards as homes
> and nurses as fathers and mothers is
> strained at several points by the fact
> that patients on "back wards" do not
> mature like children, and sometimes
> perform grossly deviant acts. This can
> cause a violent rejection of the model
> and the adoption of a more derogatory one:
> "A lot of them can't talk the same as
> animals can't. I've always maintained
> that what they want here is a vet, not
> a psychiatrist." (Jones; 1975, p.109)

Although, as I shall explain in Chapter Five, I believe Jones has misunderstood the nature of ward classifications, her report does confirm the existence, in the hospitals she studied, of classification based on terminology similar to the terminology used in the Jane Eagle hospital.

The Balderton Project team in their account of Balderton Hospital reported a similar terminology and classification. The team used the "unofficial" accounts of nurses as the basis of

the interpretive framework of their study and
therefore created an "official" account. The team
described one ward in the following way:

> physical dependence is still an important
> element in the care. But, for example,
> all patients are mobile. This is the
> lower grade of the two children's wards
> with both boys and girls living on it.
> (Dartington et al: 1973, p.4)

The project team not only used the
terminology descriptively, they also used it
analytically as in the following extract:

> Ainsdale Ward, because it is very
> difficult to categorise in terms of
> patient characteristics is the most
> complex ... We would rather see it as
> a kind of barometer of the whole hospital
> so that, when the hospital is overloaded
> with low-grade patients and Nasefield
> cannot contain all the high dependency
> males, the overflow goes to Ainsdale;
> when the nurses feel they have succeeded
> in doing sufficiently well with some of
> their higher grade patients for them to be
> relatively independent, these are taken
> from Ainsdale to the pre-discharge unit.
> (Dartington et al: 1973, pp.6-7)

These accounts show that the terminology
recorded at the Jane Eagle and reported in the
first part of this section can also be identified
in other English mental handicap hospitals and
possibly also in the U.S.A. (MacAndrew and
Edgerton: 1964). In the remainder of this
section, I shall examine official accounts of
institutions caring for the mental handicap that
can be found in historical sources. These are
official accounts. They were written public
statements not recorded verbal private
statements.

Official accounts

Contemporary hospitals for the mentally
handicapped are derived from the inter-war mental
deficiency colony. The central department
responsible for colonies in the inter-war years
was the Board of Control. The mental deficiency

colony was the centre piece of the new service. The Board not only encouraged and pressurised local mental deficiency committees to set up colonies but also provided several models for these colonies, especially in the Report of the Wood Committee (Report of the Mental Deficiency Committee: 1929) and the Departmental Committee Report (Report of the Departmental Committee: 1931).

The 1929 Wood Report used the grade classification as an organising framework for its report and for the pattern of services. Their use of terminology was not consistent but is clearly the source of the grade terminology used in contemporary hospitals. In their introduction they divided mental defectives into three main grades:

> Idiocy - This is the lowest grade of
> defect...

> Imbecility - This is the medium grade of
> defect. Imbeciles stand above the idiots
> in that they can be taught to understand
> and protect themselves from many common
> physical dangers. They stand below the
> feeble-minded, in that, whilst many of
> them can be trained to perform simple
> tasks under supervision, they are
> generally incapable of earning their
> living, or of contributing materially
> towards their keep...

> Feeble-mindedness - This is the mildest
> grade of defect... (Report of the
> Mental Deficiency Committee: 1929, Part
> 1, para.20)

In the Report the terms feeble minded and high grade tended to be used interchangeably as in the following discussion:

> We can well believe that many high-grade
> defectives would escape detection in
> those days when the problem of the
> feeble-minded was only beginning to be
> recognised. (Report of the Mental
> Deficiency Committee: 1929, Part II,
> para.85c)

The Committee used the term low grade to refer to the other grades of mental defective. However occasionally this category was subdivided into ambulant and nonambulant low grades. The nonambulant low grades were, then, referred to as cot and chair cases. For example Dr. Lewis used the term cot and chair in his investigation of the incidence of mental deficiency. He appears to have used the term rather inconsistently. He used cot and chair as a term for all nonambulant defectives (Report of the Mental Deficiency Committee: 1929, Part 4, p.127) and also referred to low grade nonambulant defectives (Report of the Mental Deficiency Committee: 1929, Part 4, pp.207-217, Tables 25-27).

The Wood Committee attached great importance to proper classification and it formed a recurrent theme in the report. They wanted to establish:

> fully equipped colonies conducted on modern lines, where adequate classification could be secured... (Report of the Mental Deficiency Committee: 1929, Part 3, p.42)

Using the Wood Committee's classification and categories it is possible to draw a diagram of the internal structure of their ideal colony. (See Diagram 3.1). A comparison of this diagram with a similar one for the Jane Eagle Hospital reveals a similarity of the classifications (See Diagram 3.3). Although Jane Eagle Hospital was planned over 30 years after the Wood Committee's Report, its internal structure was closely modelled on the ideal colony pattern, and was closer to this model than that of Balderton Hospital (Diagram 3.4). (Dartington et al: 1973, pp.3-8)

The 1931 Departmental Committee used similar terminology to the Wood Committee and identified three main classes of defective:

> Idiots (The lowest grade of defective)...
> Many of them are paralysed and have to
> be kept in special cots and chairs...
>
> Imbeciles (The medium grade of
> defective)...
>
> The Feeble-Minded (The mildest grade of
> defective) and moral defectives... Many
> have intelligence enough to resent being

associated with the lower grades.
(Report of the Departmental Committee:
1931, para.11)

The Committee concentrated on the internal
structure of the ideal colony and its model only
differed in minor details from the model outlined
in the report of the Wood Committee (See Diagram
3.2).

Comment Both unofficial accounts (records of
verbal statements) and official accounts (records
of written schemes) of mental handicap hospitals
use similar terminologies to describe and classify
wards and patients. There was a predominant grade
classification which was supplemented by age and

Diagram 3.1   Ideal colony (Wood Committee)

Age	Grade	Sex
Adult	High	Male
		Female
	Low	Male
		Female
	Cot and Chair	Male
		Female
Children	High	Male
		Female
	Low	Male
		Female

Possible Extra Wards

Difficult patients

Elderly cases

Nursery children

Adult cripples

The Classification of Wards

Diagram 3.2   <u>Complete   colony   (Departmental Committee)</u>

<u>Age</u>	<u>Grade</u>	<u>Sex</u>
Adult	Higher	Male
		Female
	Medium	Male
		Female
	Lower	Male
		Female
Mixed	Lowest	Male
		Female

Extra Wards

Troublesome patients
Adolescent
Hospital (sick ward)

Diagram 3.3   <u>Classification   at   the   Jane   Eagle Hospital</u>

<u>Age</u>	<u>Grade</u>	<u>Sex</u>
Adult	High	Male
		Female
	Low	Male
		Female
Children	High	Male
		Female
	Low	Male
		Female
Mixed	Cot and Chair	Mixed
		Mixed

Extra Wards

Young children (i.e. nursery children)

The Classification of Wards

Diagram 3.4 <u>Classification at Balderton Hospital</u>

<u>Age</u>	<u>Grade</u>	<u>Sex</u>
Adult	High	Male
		Female
	Low	Male
		Female
	Mixed	Male
		Female
Children	High	Mixed
	Low	Mixed
	Cot and Chair	Mixed

Extra Wards

Physically Ill
Elderly Cases
Adolescents

sex classifications. In the second section of this chapter, I shall use unofficial accounts, that I recorded at the Jane Eagle hospital, to identify other classifications and groupings of patients.

3.3 OTHER CLASSIFICATIONS OF PATIENTS

     The classification of patients discussed in the last section was not the only classification I recorded. When I interviewed nurses, I asked them to describe the patients in the whole hospital, in the different wards in the hospital and on the wards in which they were currently working. Each level of description was based on a classification of patients. The first section of this chapter concentrated on one level of classification. In this section I shall examine the other levels, looking at the hospital level briefly and the subward classification in more detail by concentrating on structure and function of the classification on one ward.

<u>Relationship between different levels of classification</u>
     In the last section the ward level

classification of patients was presented as an autonomous level. Indeed the first account I reported, treated it as such, by jumping straight into a discussion of the wards. However other accounts placed this discussion into context :

> Question - Why do these patients need a
> special hospital?

> Answer - They don't look after themselves
> so they've got to have someone to do it.

> Question - What causes this inability?

> Answer - Their intelligence, their low
> intelligence.

> Question - How would you describe Seagull
> and how would you say Seagull differs
> from other wards in the hospital?

> Answer - It's a much higher grade ward, much
> higher intelligence, they can do a lot
> more things for themselves.

In this account, at the first or hospital level, the patients were (implicitly) contrasted with normal people by their dependency.

> Normal : Patient :: Independent : Dependent

i.e. the difference between normal people and patients was the same as the difference between independent and dependent people. Within this overall dependency, Seagull patients were contrasted to other patients by their lower dependency. This can be represented in the following way:

> Seagull Ward : Other Wards :: Lower
> Dependency : Higher Dependency

In the following interview this type of account was developed a stage further with a third subward level.

> Question - How would you describe the
> patients to someone who knew very little
> about the hospital?

Answer - Well, I think they'd have to realise that they are all mentally subnormal. They act like children of their mental age.

Question - How do the patients on this ward (Seagull) differ from others in the hospital?

Answer - They're classed as high grade girls. They have a lot of mental disorders as well as their subnormality. They need a lot of observing. You have to try and treat them as adults.

Question - Do you think there are different sorts of patients on the ward?

Answer - Yes. The wheelchairs, then you get the old dears. They like to be on their own a bit. Then you get the Ruth type ones, the young ones, the highly strung ones "I want, I want," all the time.

If this interview is broken into its constituent parts it would read as a series of contrasts at hospital, ward and subward levels:

Normal : Patient :: Adult : Children

Seagull: Other :: Adult : Children

Old Dears : Young Ones :: Undemanding :
                                    Demanding

The ward contrasts in this account represented a different set of contrasts to the ward contrasts used by my first respondent (see the first interview in Section One). Represented in the same way that interview would have read:

High grade : Low grade : Cot and Chair ::
     Child : Animal : Vegetable

Thus the terms used do not necessarily have a constant meaning but may acquire their meaning from the context in which they are used and the explicit or implicit contrast involved.
     The analogy of a ward within a ward was

commonly used in the discussion of subward classifications. In the following account, not only was a ward name used to refer to a grouping within a ward but the groupings in the ward were based on the same principles as the classification of wards.

> Question - How do patients on this ward (Seagull) differ from others in the hospital?

> Answer - We've got three different wards here. We've got the less intelligent low grade Pelican type and our handicapped ones, our bright high grade ones who tend to be our disturbed element, like Glynis, Sarah, Anne and Carol. We've got our medium grade undisturbed, like Ethel Grimes and our old ones like Auntie. The younger more disturbed girls send the old ones up the wall. And the low grades need a lot of help in self-care toileting and washing and all this. The disturbed girls present a socialisation problem. They need a lot more taking into the community, education in social skills such as cooking.

This discussion can be in represented in a diagram (Diagram 3.5) which is similar to the ward classifications in Diagrams 3.1 - 3.4.

Diagram 3.5 <u>Classification of patients on Seagull Ward</u>

<u>Age</u>	<u>Grade</u>
Old	(Unspecified)
Young	High grade
	Medium grade
	Low grade
Mixed	Multiply Handicapped

The use of the "ward within a ward" analogy indicates that some nurses saw the ward level as the most important level of classification and

86

used it as a model for the grouping of patients within wards. The ward level had a more concrete and visible form in the separate villas. However if nurses gave primacy to the ward level this was because they gave primacy to its utility and function. The function of the ward level classification will be a major theme in the remainder of this book. In the remainder of this section I shall concentrate on the subward classification.

The subward classification on Pelican Ward

The material used in this section is derived from a long written account of the patients on a low grade ward, Pelican. The account was written specifically for the research. As Goody points out this makes this account more systematic than equivalent verbal accounts and enables the author of the account to be more explicit about the principles of her taxonomy.

> Writing gives us the opportunity for just such a monologue (based on talking freely about one's thoughts) that oral intercourse so often prevents. It enables an individual to "express" his thoughts at length, without interruption, with corrections and deletions, and according to some appropriate formula. (Goody: 1977, p.160)

The author divided her account into three parts. In the first part, she outlined her classification. In the second part, she discussed the principles behind her classification. In the third part, she discussed individual patients and their classification.

Overall classification The respondent divided the patients on Pelican Ward into five groups ranging from group one, who were totally dependent, to group five who were relatively independent.

Pelican
Classifications:
1. Patients who are totally dependent on staff, little or no self care. These patients virtually have to be carried to the toilet. (5 patients)

2.   Patients who are <u>very dependent on staff</u>,
      some independent motivation. They can
      get to the toilet by themselves as long
      as you point them in the right
      direction. (5 patients)

3.   Patients who need a lot of help from staff,
      but who have definite ideas of their own
      and a certain amount of self help.
      (2 patients)

4.   Patients who are reasonably self-reliant
      and manage to look after themselves with
      supervision but without physical
      assistance. This group contains most of
      the patients. (9 patients)

5.   Patients who are completely independent and
      who look after themselves with a greater
      or lesser degree of success. (2 patients)
      (Emphases in the original text).

<u>Principles behind the classification</u>   In
justifying her classification, the respondent
suggested that it was not the only possible
classification. She had concentrated on physical
dependency, i.e. the assistance patients needed
from staff to obtain the basic necessities of
life. She neglected the behaviour problems
presented by the patients.

      I have divided the Pelican girls into
      categories of their physical demands on
      staff because these seem to be the most
      apt on this particular ward situation.
      The mental demands of each patient do not
      necessarily correspond to the category in
      which she is placed.

The terms she used, mental and physical demands,
suggest that this is a task oriented
classification and the respondent was stressing
deficits of behaviour in terms of self help. She
was disregarding problem behaviour.

<u>Typical low grades</u>   Three of the five groups were
typically low grade, i.e. ambulant but dependent
or disturbed. One patient, Sarah, combined many
of the characteristics seen as typical of this
group - an unattractive, incompetent, difficult

girl who required physical control. The respondent
described her in the following way:

When Sarah arrived and turned out to be far
worse than anyone had anticipated things
became very unpleasant for her. She is
a demanding, aggressive, anti-social child,
also she is physically very ugly and rather
hard to like. She speaks repetitively in
phrases, in a very middle-class accent, and
she comes across as being a rather
ludicrous and pathetic imitation of what
she should be.
She was a completely disruptive influence
on the ward - refusing to comply with the
routine, i.e she would not use the toilet
if taken - retained her urine and then
went and flooded her bed. She refused to
eat - throwing her food, tables, chairs,
banging her elbows on the tables, screaming
and swearing. She kept awake at night,
often screaming and disturbing other
patients. Although it was not hard to see
why she was behaving as she was (she was an
extremely unhappy child who had obviously
loved her home), it was difficult to
sympathise with her and be tolerant as
she refused any kind of contact. I think
that initially the nursing staff did try
hard with Sarah but the more we gave, the
more demanding she became. It also puts
one in a very difficult position when other
patients see bad behaviour being rewarded
with lots of individual attention.
There is no doubt that Sarah received quite
brutal treatment when she refused to comply
with the ward routine and to integrate with
the other patients. She was hit quite
often but this served no purpose but to
make her more aggressive towards herself.
Not only did she smack herself very hard but
she refused to eat, lost a lot of weight and
became physically very ill. She also
started to have a great number of epileptic
fits and she became a physical and mental
problem patient.
Her parents both complained on every visit
about her clothes and the state of her
health and this was all taken out on Sarah.
Everybody disliked her even more.

Atypical patients In addition to the typical
low grade groups, the respondent identified two
atypical groups - patients whose physical
handicaps made them more like cot and chair
patients and patients whose greater social
competence made them more like high grade
patients. There were two patients in the
high grade group. One had been difficult to
manage on Seagull, the high grade ward for women,
and had been transferred to Pelican. The other,
Rosemary, had been admitted from another hospital.
Rosemary's case indicates how the nurses were
willing and able to manipulate the classification
of wards. Rosemary should have been on Seagull
Ward but she was useful on Pelican Ward. Her
position was described in the following way:

> Rosemary tends to treat the other patients
> with an air of bored superiority. She has
> as little as possible to do with them except
> in the course of her work. She tends to be
> domineering and intolerant. At night she
> undresses the other patients and puts out
> their morning clothes. Whether she has been
> made responsible for this or has made her-
> self responsible I don't know. The lower
> grade patients bear the brunt of Rosemary's
> bad moods. She will tend to let anyone, who
> through general slowness or inability
> irritates her, have it. She does not make
> punishing other patients a habitual
> occupation but if she has been crossed over
> anything the other patients will suffer for
> it ...
> It must be very difficult to regard oneself
> as the only sane person in a crowd of
> people of extremely restricted ability.
> She has no social contact with the others
> as there's no-one capable of sustaining any
> sort of relationship at her level.

In a conversation between two nurses about
Rosemary, there was a clear emphasis on her
atypical position and on the exploitation of her
behaviour. (Nurse N was the author of the
classification discussed above.)

> Nurse N. I went to a party on Pelican this
> afternoon. It was awful. It was
> Rosemary Barker's birthday party and she

really stuck out like a sore thumb. She
was all nicely dressed and her hair was
all done and she had to have it with all
those slobbering low grades. Why don't
they move her to Seagull?

Nurse J. It's the old "top dog" argument.
They're keeping her on Pelican because
she's happiest as "top dog" on Pelican.
I've never trusted that "top dog"
argument. The real reason they're
keeping her is that she is a good worker
and they don't want to lose her. She
makes all the beds in the morning.

At a case conference Rosemary's position on
the ward was questioned by the social worker.
However the consultant and ward nurses formed an
alliance to keep Rosemary on the ward.

Clinical Psychologist - I didn't test
Rosemary but Mrs F. (another Psychologist)
did ... on that performance she was as
high as anyone else in the hospital.
Higher than any of the patients on Magpie
(high grade ward) but there are probably
a few on Seagull (high grade ward) that
are higher.

Social Worker - Is Rosemary suitably placed
on Pelican (low grade ward)?

Ward Consultant - We have talked about the
possibility of transferring Rosemary to
Seagull. It was difficult to assess her
at her previous hospital because we only
saw her for about five minutes amongst
30 other patients. She seems to have
settled down well on Pelican and she has
got her own room which she takes great
pride in. If she is transferred to
Seagull it won't be possible to give her
her own room. I don't think she will hit
it off with the elite on Seagull. There
are three or four girls on Seagull that
do their own jobs and Rosemary will be
upset because they will not allow her to
do her own jobs. Is Rosemary sociable
on the ward?

91

Staff Nurse - She tends to keep herself to herself and does not mix with the other patients. She will help look after some of the other patients if asked.

Social Worker - Is this because there are no other patients of her type on Pelican, they are all on Seagull.

Staff Nurse - She refuses to mix with the Seagull girls.

Ward Consultant - In view of the fact that Rosemary has only just arrived at the Jane Eagle, I think she should remain where she is.

This type of manipulation of the patient classification has been recorded in other English mental handicap hospitals.

Staff actually used the relationship between patients to serve their own ends. Thus a number of patients of higher ability were employed as "domestics" in the villas, and these often came to take a considerable power over the patients in the villa. (Tyne: 1974, p.73)

Comment This classification of patients on Pelican was designed with a specific purpose in mind - to provide information about the physical needs of the patients. The subward groupings indicated that the nurses exploited the classification to facilitate their work. The patients on Pelican could be divided into two groups - typical low grade patients and atypical patients. The atypical patients were seen as either cot and chair patients or high grade patients. They were on the ward either because they were useful or because they were a nuisance on other wards. The presence of atypical patients therefore represented power relations between the nurses in different wards - either the ability to get rid of problem patients or the ability to retain useful patients.

3.4 CONCLUSION

In this chapter I have identified three

separate levels of patient classification at the
Jane Eagle Hospital, hospital, ward and subward
classifications. The ward level had a physical,
visible and permanent form, the villas. It was
therefore the most consistent. Equivalent
classifications could be identified in other
unofficial and official accounts of hospitals for
the mentally handicapped. The physical visibility
of the wards and the general agreement about
terminology meant that nurses tended to take the
classification of wards for granted. The general
agreement meant there was less discussion of and
speculation about the ward classification and it
was more difficult to understand the function and
meaning of the ward classification. In contrast
since there was less agreement about subward
classifications, nurses discussed these
classifications more and the purpose of each
classification was more obvious.

CHAPTER 4
THE MEANING OF THE CLASSIFICATION OF PATIENTS:
MIXTURES AND ANOMALIES

4.1 INTRODUCTION

In Chapter Two, I discussed the difficulty of
making explicit aspects of reality that
participants take for granted. The subward
classification did not present this difficulty.
Since each subward classification was ad hoc and
for a specific purpose, the respondents were often
aware and could usually make explicit their
criteria of classification. However the ward
classification was treated as self-evident. It
was not designed or formulated by any of the staff
at the hospital but by the committee which
designed the hospital and even they were
constrained by precedents. Thus existing staff
accepted it as a fact of life. They tended to use
it rather than talk about it.
As a system, the classification had both
a meaning and a purpose. Its meaning was what it
said about the individuals it classified - the
implicit information it contained. Its purpose
was the function it served for the staff and the
ways in which it related to social actions. My
problem was to understand the meaning and function
of the classification. The work of Douglas
provided a way of examining the underlying and
implicit assumptions of the patient
classification. Douglas has argued that
classifications are ways of creating order by
putting things in their right place. However
classifications are never completely successful.
There are always bits that do not fit, anomalies,
and bits that are always getting out of place,
dirt (Douglas: 1966). Douglas has suggested that
anomalies and dirt attract special interest:

94

> In <u>Purity and Danger</u> ... I argued that
> to classify is a necessary human
> activity and that there is a universal
> human tendency to pass adverse judgement
> on that which eludes classification or
> refuses to fit into the tidy
> compartments of the mind. (Douglas: 1975,
> pp.284-285)

She modified her position to suggest that
anomalies and dirt have a symbolic potential, and
the exploitation of this potential depends on the
social context, i.e. the type of social relations
that need to be expressed in symbolic form. I
shall return to the type of relationship encoded
in the classification in Chapter Seven. At this
stage I am more interested in the principles of
taxonomy. Anomalies and dirt, the bits that are
out of place, draw attention to these principles
of taxonomy. They emphasise these principles by
their breach of them. Douglas used this approach
when discussing the dietary rules of the
Israelites. In Leviticus certain animals are
classified as unclean and therefore inedible.
Douglas analysed the list in the following way:

> in general the underlying principle of
> cleanness in animals is that they shall
> conform fully to their class. Those
> species are unclean which are imperfect
> members of their class, or whose class
> itself confounds the general scheme of
> the world. (Douglas: 1966, p.55)

By concentrating on unclean animals Douglas was
able to isolate the principles underlying the
classification of animals as clean or proper.

> Thus anything in the water which has not
> fins and scales is unclean ... Nothing
> is said about predatory habits or
> scavenging. The only sure test for
> cleanness in a fish is its scales and
> its propulsion by means of fins.
> (Douglas: 1966, p.55)

The same approach can be applied to the
classification of wards at the Jane Eagle.
Although, in theory, each ward should be
homogeneous, in practice, there was some mixing

e.g. high grade (Seagull) patients on a low grade ward (Pelican). In practice there were always patients in the wrong place. These inconsistencies tended to be denied and these denials contained information about the expected consequences of mixing different sorts of patients. Read in reverse the expected consequences provided information about the defining characteristics of each class of patients. There was another major inconsistency in the classification. One ward, Hawk, was consistently omitted from classifications. It defied classification and somehow cut across the different classes. An examination of the way in which Hawk ward defied classification provides further information about the defining characteristics of the classes.

The approach I will use in the first three sections of this chapter to reveal perceptions of the characteristics of each category is to examine accounts of the problems created by mixing patients from different categories. I showed in the last chapter that there were three separate modes of classification in the groupings of wards, classification by grade (high grade, low grade and cot and chair), classification by sex (male and female) and classification by age (child and adult). Therefore there are three ways of mixing patients. Different grades, different sexes or different age groups can be mixed. Staff believed that each type of mixture created its own problems and I shall consider each in turn.

4.2 MIXING GRADES

There were three ways of mixing two grades - cot and chair patients could be mixed with low grade patients, cot and chair patients with high grade patients or low grade patients with high grade patients. Each mixture was seen as creating its own special problems and therefore provides information about the perceived characteristics of the patients mixed. I shall deal with each mix in turn.

Cot and chair and low grade

My first statement is based on a discussion by a ward consultant of a mixture of all the patients. In it, he stressed the vulnerability of cot and chair patients and the aggressiveness of low grade patients.

> We are trying to group patients according
> to age and handicap ... Kushlick (who
> advocates mixed or cross sectional units)
> would have great problems in introducing a
> sectorised system in a whole region. Each
> unit would have to contain a total cross-
> section of all patients e.g. Ravensbourn
> (cot and chair), Magpie (high grade) and
> Kestrel (low grade) patients all on the
> same unit. This is impossible as it would
> mean that Graham Wells (a low grade
> Kestrel patient) would destroy the
> Ravensbourn patients. Either a
> classification of patients would creep
> in or else Graham Wells would be sent to
> Rampton (a special hospital).

Cot and chair and high grade

The consultant did not see the high grades as
a risk to the safety of the vulnerable
cot and chair patients. Indeed other statements
indicated a threat in the other direction. Mixing
high grade and cot and chair patients could retard
the development of high grade patients.

> The hospital is laid out on a villa
> system by which all units are an
> independent body apart from the doctors,
> the nursing officers and the kitchen
> staff.
>
> Question - So the place is split into
> wards?
>
> Answer - Yes, depending on their
> capabilities, mental age, sex, degree of
> subnormality.
>
> Question - Do you think this is a good
> system dividing them up in this way?
>
> Answer - Yes.
>
> Question - What are the advantages?
>
> Answer - Well if all the wards were mixed up
> then I think that the patients that had
> the higher grade of subnormality would

97

> in fact regress because they'd be put with
> the people like the kids on Ravensbourn.
> I should say it's very depressing for
> another patient to come here
> (Ravensbourn).

Although the cot and chair patients were seen as a threat to the social development of high grade patients, cot and chair wards were seen as safe environments for elderly patients who were no longer a risk to the vulnerable cot and chair patients and who were themselves at risk on the ambulant wards. During my field work at the Jane Eagle hospital, a geriatric unit was created on one of the cot and chair wards mainly for patients from the two high grade wards. I shall discuss this case more fully in the section on the mixing of age groups.

High grade and low grade

Again it was the high grade patients who were expected to suffer from the contact. Their greater social sensibilities were affronted by the anti-social behaviour of low grade patients. The following statement was taken from a discussion of a placement of a low grade patient, Pippa, on a high grade ward, Seagull:

> Pippa is totally out of place on here
> (Seagull). She is always wet and dirty.
> She is noisy as well. It is unfair on
> the other girls. She should really be
> on Pelican (a low grade ward). Look
> at her. She's just had a clean dress
> on and she still stinks of urine and
> is covered with vomit.

High grade wards were occasionally used as safe environments for low grade patients. For example one of the patients transferred from Magpie (high grade ward) to the new geriatric unit on Ravensbourn (cot and chair ward) had originally been transferred from Kestrel (low grade ward) to Magpie following an incident in which his eye was destroyed.

Low grade wards could be used as refractory wards for difficult high grades. The use of low grade wards for difficult high grades is discussed in the following extract:

The ward system in subnormality hospitals
is fairly arbitrary, I've had this
problem with Adam Greatchild.
Intelligence-wise he's a typical Leopard
(high grade) patient but he's a totally
disruptive patient on the ward. For
example, with the T.V. set - he's
constantly pushing it over and breaking
it. Eventually I had to decide which I
was going to put first, the interests of
Adam or the interests of the other boys.
So I applied to have Adam transferred to
Drake, where they were better equipped to
deal with Adam's disruptive behaviour.
Their T.V. is protected by a special
wooden box. I've been accused of palming
off my problem patients on to other wards
but that's not the case at all, because
I've kept two of the most difficult,
Toby Jacks and Mark Stevens.

Discussion

In their discussions of the problems of
mixing grades staff tended to emphasise the
following characteristics:

1. Cot and chair patients were seen as
physically vulnerable and fairly passive. Their
ward was seen as a suitable environment for other
patients who had become (through old age)
physically vulnerable and passive.

2. Low grade patients were seen as
physically active but anti-social. Their ward was
seen as a suitable environment for other patients
with difficult or problem behaviour.

3. High grade patients were seen as socially
aware. Although their ward was not as safe as a
cot and chair ward, it was seen as safer than the
low grade wards.

4.3 MIXING SEXES

Sexual behaviour is a form of behaviour that
attracts considerable social attention. Most
societies devote considerable energy to
controlling and channelling sexual behaviour as it
is the basis of the reproduction of social groups.
In many societies the control of reproduction is a

group concern and closely connected with the
political and economic relations of groups.
Marriage is not only a relationship established
between individuals but also a relationship
between groups and frequently involves a complex
exchange of material and symbolic goods. This is
a central theme in social anthropology (see for
example Levi-Strauss: 1969 and Needham: 1971).
Douglas has suggested that these exchanges have an
important impact not only on the way these
cultures organise their social relations but also
on the way they classify their natural universe.

> The boundaries of the categories of nature
> are expected to show a parallel with
> the inclusions and rejections permitted
> on social boundaries. Where society is
> based on the structuring of birth and
> marriage, the most significant exchanges
> will concern transfers of women. (Douglas:
> 1975, p.296)

Our society is not based on the structuring
of birth and marriage and therefore marriage and
child birth is generally considered an individual
and private responsibility as long as the
individuals concerned are competent adults.
However incompetence, usually implied by a
dependent status such as childhood, brings into
play a whole set of collective and public
considerations. To understand the information
provided by division of sexes we need to consider
these public considerations and the way they have
affected the organisation of mental handicap
hospitals.

Sex and the Mentally Handicapped

The current legal and administrative
framework for the mentally handicapped can be
traced back to the Radnor Commission (Report of
the Royal Commission: 1908) and the 1913 Mental
Deficiency Act. The general social and political
context of the Commission and the Act was one of
crisis and class conflict. The response of the
Liberal Administration was the so called Liberal
Reforms. Hay has suggested that reforms, such as
the National Insurance Act of 1911 had a double
objective, to win over the industrious poor and to
exclude the idle and degenerate residuum (Hay:
1975, p.34). The internal class conflict and

external imperial tensions made the issue of reproduction of the population a public and political issue. The Boer War had drawn attention to the poor health status of the population. A response to these various pressures was a movement towards increased collective control of reproduction which was articulated by the Eugenics Movement. The movement sought to increase the reproduction of the more able and reduce the reproduction of the less able in society.

The Eugenics Society derived its intellectual base from studies which claimed to show the inheritance of intellectual ability (Galton: 1869) and defect (Dugdale: 1910) and the higher fertility rates of mental defectives (Goddard: 1931). During the 1890's the lower ability group were labelled feeble minded and the first steps were made to control their reproduction. For example the Lancashire and Cheshire Society for the Permanent Care of the Feeble Minded established the Sandlebridge Colony near Manchester for the lifelong segregation of the feeble minded. Mary Dendy, a key member of the society, argued that "only permanent care can be really efficacious in stemming the great level of feebleness of mind in our country" (Dendy: 1920).

The various societies for the care of the feeble minded and the Eugenics Society played an important part in the appointment of the Radnor Commission and had an important influence on its report and in the subsequent campaign to implement the recommendations of the Commission. The Commission endorsed the views of campaigners. It accepted that mental defect was hereditary and that defectives were fertile. It recommended that the reproduction of defectives should be controlled by institutional care.

> In conclusion, we may fairly sum up the general effect of the evidence as follows:
> (1) That both on the grounds of fact and of theory there is the highest degree of probability that "feeble-mindedness" is usually spontaneous in origin - that is not due to influence acting on the parent - and tends strongly to be inherited.
> (2) That, especially in view of the

evidence concerning fertility, the
prevention of mentally defective persons
from becoming parents would tend largely
to diminish the number of such persons in
the population.
(3)   That the evidence for these conclusions
strongly supports measures ... for
placing mentally defective persons, men
and women, who are living at large and
uncontrolled, in institutions where they
will be employed and detained; and in
this, and in other ways, kept under
effectual supervision so long as may be
necessary. (The Royal Commission: 1908,
para.553)

Initial legislative proposals by the Liberal
Administration included a fairly broad attempt to
control   the   reproduction   of   defectives.
Individuals were to be committed to an institution
if they were defectives:

in whose case it is desirable in the
interests of the community that they
should be deprived of the opportunity
of procreating children. (Leach: 1913,
p.iv)

Opponents of the legislation succeeded in limiting
this to high grade female defectives who were:

in the receipt of poor relief at the time
of giving birth to an illegitimate child
or when pregnant of such child. (Leach:
1913, p.9)

The   prevention of   the   reproduction   of
high grade defectives became an accepted part of
policy. The Board of Control regularly discussed
the issue in its annual reports and commended
different measures to local mental deficiency
committees.   The   Wood Committee accepted the
basic assumptions of the Royal Commission and
extended them to a group which they referred to as
"subnormal". This category included not only all
existing   defectives   but all   other   "social
inefficients" of marginal intelligence. The Wood
Committee endorsed the practice of institutional
segregation   as   a   method   of   controlling
defectives:

the relative fertility of this (subnormal)
group is greater than that of normal
persons. In point of fact the disparity
in the actual as opposed to the potential
fertility of the normal and the subnormal
sections of the population is increasing,
the families of the subnormal groups
remaining as large as hitherto while those
of the better social groups are steadily
diminishing in size. Sterilization,
segregation and even the more moderate
remedial measure of the regulation of
marriage (are all possible remedies).
(Mental Deficiency Committee: 1929,
Part 3, p.82)

The Departmental Committee on sterilization
advocated voluntary sterilization as an
alternative to institutional segregation
(Departmental Committee: 1934, para.103).

Sex and the internal structure of institutions
Since one major objective of mental
deficiency colonies was the prevention of sexual
reproduction and the colonies were modelled on
lunatic asylums, colonies were designed to
separate the sexes, amongst both staff and
patients. Either two separate institutions were
constructed or the institution was divided into a
female "side" and a male "side". The history of
mental handicap hospitals shows the gradual
breaking down of the rigid demarcation with mixing
of staff and some mixing of patients. The areas
in which this process has proceeded the furthest
and fastest provides interesting information on
the perceived characteristics of the different
groups of patients.
The breakdown had already started in the
Departmental Report on the construction of
colonies. The Report suggested that in the case
of cot and chair patients there was little danger
of mixing sexes.

(these cases) require the constant attention
normally given to infants and, indeed,
they are mostly just as helpless... Both
sexes could thus be accommodated in one
block until such time as an increase in
numbers rendered a new block necessary.
(Departmental Committee: 1931, p.20)

Their attitude to cot and chair cases contrasted strongly with their attitude to other patients, especially adults.

> The administrative buildings should form
> a barrier between the home (sic) for adult
> patients of different sexes.
> (Departmental Committee: 1931, p.21)

At the Jane Eagle hospital the breakdown could also be observed. The hospital was planned in the early 1960s and followed the Board of Control model closely. The original plans showed a central administrative block dividing the hospital into a male side and a female side. An area at the top of the site was designated "male recreation area" and an equivalent area at the bottom "female recreation area". The majority of the male wards were still on the "male side" and all the female wards on the "female side". All the wards on the "male side" had urinals in the patients' toilets, whereas none of the wards on the "female side" had these. Diagram 3.3 indicates that the wards for the younger and less able patients tended to be mixed whereas those for the older more able patients were still segregated. Diagram 3.4 indicates that the process had gone a stage further at Balderton Hospital, where all the children's wards were mixed. It is now more acceptable for the mentally handicapped to have sexual relations and there is no longer the same public concern about controlling reproduction. However the staff of mental handicap hospitals have retained a more "traditional" attitude towards the sexual activities of patients and the mixing of sexes has only occurred in areas of minimum risk.

The sexual behaviour of the mentally handicapped
I have already shown that cot and chair patients were not considered by the Departmental Committee to be a sexual risk. This is still the case and all cot and chair wards at the Jane Eagle were mixed.
In the last section I argued that nurses viewed the behaviour of low grade patients as anti-social. Their sexual behaviour was seen in the same way. It was not seen as purposeful or collectively oriented, i.e. heterosexual and oriented towards procreation, but as physical and

individual, i.e. autoerotism or masturbation. A ward consultant described the arrival of a group of low grade patients in the following way:

> I tell them (visitors from other hospitals)
> that if you have been here (Kestrel Ward)
> five years ago you would not have
> recognised these patients. It was a
> nightmare. On the first of February 1966
> twenty five half naked incontinent
> masturbating patients were dumped here.
> It was a seething mass of idiocy.

Staff reacted with horror when such behaviour was exploited by the more competent. One low grade patient, referred to by the staff as "Saliva", was admitted to the hospital pregnant. The pregnancy, which was terminated, was described by one nurse in the following way:

> It's absolutely unthinkable. How could
> anybody do it to her. She's a mass of
> saliva, vomit and urine.

The sexual behaviour of high grade patients was seen as a problem, both in the sense that it was purposeful and socially oriented and in the sense that it was difficult to control. The following extract is taken from the aide-memoire used by a student nurse when conducting visitors round the hospital.

> Magpie is where the highest grade adult
> male patients reside ... Seagull is the
> high grade adult female ward. Magpie and
> Seagull are run on about the same lines
> and between them they probably present the
> biggest problems (management wise) than
> any of the other wards, as the higher
> grade patients present management problems
> that you don't come across with the lower
> grade patients, such as sexual problems,
> social problems. Some of them would be
> able to live in hostels in the community
> and they are aware of this. This can
> cause problems in the ward situation when
> these individuals become frustrated with
> the hospital environment.

Discussion

Examination of the classification of wards by sex provides further information about the characteristics of different grades of patient. Cot and chair patients of different sexes could be mixed. They were seen as passive, i.e. deficient in behaviour including sexual behaviour. The classification could be relaxed for low grades, especially low grade children. Their sexual behaviour was seen as physical and individualistic not social or collective. Masturbation was seen as unpleasant but not as dangerous within the hospital. However they were potentially at risk from sexual exploitation by the more competent. The sexual behaviour of the high grades was seen as both social and purposeful. It created a problem of control.

4.4 MIXING AGE GROUPS

There is some evidence that policy makers feel that different age groups should not be mixed. The Peggy Jay Committee found it unacceptable that children should live in mental handicap hospitals (Committee of Enquiry: 1979, para.111). Hospital staff found it quite acceptable that mentally handicapped children should live in hospital, indeed they seemed to be more concerned about the young upsetting the old.

The young upsetting the old

All adult wards had a mixture of young and old patients. This was seen as a minor problem. On the high grade ward the emphasis was on social disruption created by the younger patients.

> The older patients present the greatest problem on the ward. It's too noisy for them. The younger patients aggravate them.

One nurse suggested as a solution that the ward should be divided into units, one for the old and one for the young.

> You have the old dears, they like to be on their own. Then you have the young ones, the highly strung ones. There's quite a variety but they seem to get on O.K. ...
> Occasionally if it gets too noisy, the

old ones tend to take themselves off.
This is one of the things I'd definitely
like to change. I'd definitely like to
section off this ward so that you'd got
different wards. A quiet ward for the
older ones.

On low grade wards, the younger patients were
seen as a physical threat to the older patients.
The following extract from Trevor Eave's case
conference indicates the dangers of a low grade
ward and the use of the cot and chair ward as a
safe refuge.

He is a low grade mongol... Trevor is a
timid and frightened person and is very
afraid of being knocked over ... It was
felt, as Trevor is so small, frail and
timid, he might gain more confidence in a
calmer and less mobile environment. When
the Geriatric Unit at Ravensbourn is ready
this would be the most suitable place for
him.

Age, grade and development

It might appear to be strange to mix the
youngest and least able patients (cot and chair)
with the oldest and most able (elderly high grade)
patients but staff perceived similarities between
the two groups. Both groups were seen as
relative.y passive and both groups were expected
to deteriorate. The following extract comes from
a discussion of a proposed restructuring of wards.
One of the two cot and chair wards in the
hospital (Beaver Ward) was to move into the villa
used by Seagull patients to be nearer the new
patients' school. The respondent was concerned
about the patients on the other cot and chair
ward, Ravensbourn.

Question - So there was going to be a
graduation with the best cot and chair on
the new Seagull and the worst up here
(Ravensbourn)?

Answer - Yes ... We (Ravensbourn nurses)
opposed it mainly because of working on
that type of ward. Originally they
weren't going to have geriatrics up here -
they were going to Beaver. They were

going to have some geriatrics along with
heavily handicapped. Now we were going to
have all the older and heavily handicapped
up here - ones that don't go anywhere and
we opposed it because you'd never get
nurses to work properly on that type of
ward because it is so monotonous and
boring ... You don't get any of the
interesting ones, they (the older and the
heavily handicapped) just go downhill
anyway.

In contrast to the pessimism about
elderly patients, there was optimism about
the development of the youngest patients, even on
the cot and chair wards , as in the following
interview:

Question - So your objective is to improve
the patient inside the hospital?

Answer - Try and improve. Yes.

Question - How far do you think you really
stand a chance of success with this?

Answer - On Ravensbourn?

Question - Yes.

Answer - Some I think are capable, most not.

Question - Who?

Answer - Stuart West. He's 4. He's not
reached his peak yet. He's very much
below his physical age. He's 4 and he's
got time to improve and I believe with
attention he could do lots of things.
Well he'll be out of his wheelchair for
a start. He'd be walking. He would be
feeding himself if only there was the
time to be devoted to it. If a lot of
the others had received the same attention
during childhood, then they would have a
higher standard.

The association between age and development
is a common one in our society. In the mental
handicap hospital there is a complementary

association between grade and development. High grade patients were seen as having potential for development, even discharge.

Question - What are the highest wards in the hospital?

Answer - Magpie and Seagull.

Question - What is the difference between the patients on the highest ward and on the lowest?

Answer - Well on the lowest, they are physically handicapped as well as mentally handicapped. On Seagull and Magpie there are probably only two or three that are in wheelchairs. The ones that aren't in wheelchairs are capable or could be capable of being rehabilitated and going to a hostel where they may go to a training centre by day and lead a sheltered life. Not necessarily sheltered. A lot of the lads from Magpie go down to the pub at night. They are capable of going on their own, having a pint and getting some cigarettes and coming back.

Both grade and age affected staff expectations of patient development and the two could be linked in a single model of development. Normal development is often seen as a cycle with three distinct phases: an initial period of development during childhood; a period of mature, fully socialised adulthood, and finally a periodof physical and mental deterioration into senility and death. The nurses saw different grades as diverging in different ways from this "normal" pattern. "High grades" diverged the least. Their development was seen as slower and they did not achieve full adult status. "Low grades" were seen as diverging more, with normal physical development but limited mental and social development. Cot and chair patients were seen as diverging the most, with extremely limited physical and mental development and early and often rapid deterioration.

The relationship between age, grade and staff expectations can be summarised in a diagram. In diagram 4.1 staff expectations are dichotomised into positive, plus sign, and likely to deteriorate, minus sign.

Diagram 4.1 <u>Nurses' expectations of patients</u>

	High Grade	Low Grade	Cot and chair
Elderly	−	−	−
Adult	+	−	−
Child	+	+	−

<u>Age, grade, development and ward environment.</u>
     Staff perceptions of development were associated with their perceptions of the suitable ward environment for patients. The socially oriented, potentially developing but childlike high grade patients were seen as needing a relaxed homelike environment. The objectives of nurses on Magpie Ward were described by one nurse as follows:

> The principle behind this ward is to
> make it as homely an atmosphere as
> possible in a hospital. What you try and
> achieve is not a ward at all but a home
> for the boys to come home to when they've
> been to work (i.e. at the adult training
> centre or occupational therapy department)
> all day.

     At the other extreme of the ability range, the passive cot and chair patients were not seen as responding to their environment, therefore this environment was optional. Whereas respondents described suitable environments for other grades they were silent about the environment needed by cot and chair patients.

> Answer - Parents just can't manage these
> (Ravensbourn) patients. These are in here
> till the day they die and that is it and
> you just nurse them till they do.

> Question - What keeping them clean and
> comfortable?

> Answer - Yes, and playing with them but it's

about that isn't it?

Question - What would you describe your own
job as?

Answer - I don't know really, I enjoy it.
I'm here for the patients not anything
else, I mean I'm here for the money like
everybody else but the patients come first
but the thing is on here you can't really
do a lot with them except play with them.

The active potentially violent low grade
patients were seen as having had little
development potential. At the best they could be
reduced to a fairly passive state. They were seen
as requiring a fairly tough environment, both
indestructible and rigorous.

Kestrel ... is occupied by low grade adult
men ... In the past these patients ...
were the most disturbed and aggressive
in the hospital. If you take a look back
... five to six years ago almost all the
patients were on enormous doses of drugs.
It would be nothing out of the ordinary
on a normal day, for three to four windows
to be smashed, items of furniture to be
damaged or ruined, patients injuring each
other or themselves or becoming involved
in scuffles with the staff. Under the
strict and constant supervision of the
charge nurse, who brought about and
maintained the improvement, from being
the patients who present ... the biggest
problem in the hospital they have now,
through constant supervision, observation
and habit training, been brought to the
stage where they can be managed easily
by the right staff. Under the right
conditions this ward is one of the
quietest and most peaceful in the
hospital.

Compared to other wards, low grade wards were
relatively devoid of luxuries such as decorations,
carpets and personalised clothing. Even the
parents commented on this. The following
statement was recorded in Pelican Ward Report
Book:

111

S. Painter returned from leave c/o Father.
Dr. Painter was most disgusted with the
ward because he could not find lockers
or pictures by the bed. He also wanted to
write to the Hospital Secretary in the
presence of Dr. L. (ward consultant). He
went so far as to say they must live like
"animals".

Discussion

Although nursing staff are not completely
pessimistic about patient development, pessimism
undoubtedly outweighed optimism. Belknap in his
analysis of staff attitudes in an American
Mental Hospital argued that attendants' attitudes
toward patients played an important part in their
treatment. He suggested these attitudes were
overwhelmingly negative. The attendants believed
that patients were unresponsive to treatment
(Belknap: 1956). At the Jane Eagle, staff
expectations varied according to the age and grade
of the patient. The younger and the higher the
grade of the patients, the more optimistic were
the staff. Staff perception of suitable
environments for the patients were related to
their perception of development. High grade
patients, with the greatest potential, needed a
homelike environment. Low grade patients, with
minimal potential, needed a tough environment. The
environment of cot and chair patients was of
little importance since they had little
developmental potential.

4.5 HAWK WARD: AN ANOMALY

Hawk Ward did not fit into the dominant
classification. Respondents generally did not
discuss it with the other wards. Hawk was
atypical in a number of respects. It did not look
like the other wards. The building which it
occupied, was originally planned as a small sick
unit. There were only 7 patients on the ward.
However the most important factor in its anomalous
position was its age and grade composition. All
the other wards were in theory homogeneous in
grade but mixed in age. The categories child and
adult both covered very broad age ranges. Hawk
Ward was relatively homogeneous in age but mixed
in grade, it had young children of mixed
abilities.

Hawk Ward had its own routine, characterised by intensive training. Unlike other patients, Hawk patients did not go to a therapy unit or school, the school came to them. The anomalous status of the ward was related to distinctive attitudes amongst the nurses towards development of the Hawk patients. Nurses were usually optimistic about the developmental potential of Hawk patients, however this optimism was tinged with a note of caution. Nurses had not fully decided, they were waiting to see. The headmistress of the patients' school was optimistic when she described the current position of the Hawk children.

> The Hawk children (pause) we have to send a teacher down there, that's because we haven't got a room for them in the school. When Hawk opened we just did not have one more room in the school but luckily they do form a very coherent group because the very reason they are on Hawk they're small, they are young children, they're trainable children. They're not physically handicapped ... if they get a bit older and they still remain on Hawk they come up to the school. We've got two that come up to school and they fit into the younger school group up here.

The headmistress was not totally accurate in her discussion of the current situation. Although two Hawk patients did attend the high grade group at the school (the School Group), a third Hawk patient attended the low grade group (the Playgroup). When the headmistress discussed the future of the Hawk patients she was less optimistic.

> The "B" stream (low grade) could have the odd child from Hawk who turned out as they grew older to be a bit more difficult or less likely to conform to a group. This is where it is so bad. They can transfer from Hawk to the group we call the Playgroup, which sounds as though they are going downwards. We must really try and find a new name (for the Playgroup).

113

The problem was more than one of names. No name could conceal that in transferring from the Hawk group to the Playgroup the child was being "written off" and was moving from the category of trainable to that of untrainable.

Discussion

Although Hawk was distinctive in a number of ways, the most important anomaly seemed to be its unclear status in terms of grade. Although staff were overtly optimistic about development of the Hawk children, they were also waiting to see how these children developed and what grade they fell in. The medical staff utilised this situation by using the ward as an assessment unit for children living at home.

4.6 CONCLUSION

This examination of the problems that hospital staff anticipated from mixing different groups of patients has highlighted the characteristics that nurses associated with each grade of patients and therefore one aspect of the meaning of the grade classification of patients.

High grade patients were seen as physically active and their behaviour was socially oriented. Thus their behaviour was amenable to social control. They could be useful as workers on low grade wards. They had the capacity to engage in purposeful sexual behaviour and this created a problem of control. They diverged least from the pattern of normal development but they were slow to develop, and they did not achieve full independent adult status. Since they were responsive to their environment and not wantonly destructive, efforts were made to provide high grade patients with a homelike environment.

Low grade patients were seen as anti-social, physically active and potentially dangerous. They were a danger to themselves and other patients and destroyed their environment. They had sexual behaviour but, like all their behaviour, it was not socially oriented. It was physical and individualistic. Therefore low grade patients were seen as needing physical/mechanical control; a rigid routine and a barren tough environment. Thus low grade wards could be used as refractory wards. Low grade patients diverged quite considerably from the normal model of development. Physically they developed normally but they showed little mental or social development. Thus their behaviour was always seen as behaviour and never as social action. They never attain "adulthood", i.e. a state of social independence.

Cot and chair patients were seen as passive and physically vulnerable. Their ward could therefore be used as a safe refuge for other physically vulnerable patients. Their physical handicaps limited their range of movement and they exhibited little purposive behaviour. They diverged the most from the model of normal development. They showed little physical, mental or social development and often showed an early and rapid deterioration. A lot of staff stimulation could produce some development but few staff felt it was worthwhile providing this stimulation. Since cot and chair patients were seen as relatively uninfluenced by their environment, this environment could be used in a purely functional way.

Hawk Ward was anomalous in various ways. It was smaller and it looked different. It could not be classified in grade terms. Although staff were overtly optimistic about the children's development they were also waiting to see. The anomalous position of Hawk was associated with a distinctive routine and a distinctive ward environment.

CHAPTER 5
THE MEANING OF THE CLASSIFICATION OF PATIENTS:
ORGANIC ANALOGIES

5.1   INTRODUCTION

In Chapter Four I examined the implicit
assumptions behind the ward classification of
patients by examining the problems that staff
anticipated from mixing different types of
patients and by examining the characteristics of
one anomalous ward. In this chapter I develop the
analysis of the meaning of the classification by
examining in detail one set of analogies
associated with the grade classification.

Researchers in the UK and the US have
commented on the use of organic analogies for
patients in long stay institutions for the
physically disabled, mentally ill and mentally
handicapped. The staff of long stay institutions
sometimes refer to patients as "animals" or
"vegetables". Researchers have usually been
shocked and horrified by these references and have
argued that the staff are making mistakes, i.e.
are failing to differentiate between a human being
and an animal. From this evidence researchers have
tended to argue that the staff are treating
patients as animals and that there is a simple
relationship between a set of ideas (as embodied
in verbal statements) and a pattern of actions. In
other words when staff refer to patients as
animals, they treat them as animals.

I shall argue in this chapter that
researchers have tended to misunderstand the
meaning of the statements they have recorded.
They have argued that when staff refer to patients
as animals they are mistaking them for animals and
therefore treat them as animals. I shall argue
that this misunderstanding arises from two

116

sources, an inadequate conceptualisation of the ideas involved and an associated failure to examine in detail the relationship between ideas and actions.

In Chapter Three I presented evidence that some nurses at the Jane Eagle Hospital also used organic analogies and that when high grade patients were referred to as "children", then low grade patients were referred to as "animals" and cot and chair patients were referred to as "vegetables". In this chapter I shall argue that these terms were used metaphorically and staff did not mean that certain patients were children, animals or vegetables. The meaning of the analogies was more complex than this.

In the next section of this chapter I shall examine in more detail the analyses put forward by other researchers. In the second section, I shall reexamine my evidence to see how well it fits these analyses. In the third section I shall look at an alternative explanation by examining historical sources. In the fourth Section I shall comment in more detail on the meaning and function of these analogies.

5.2 THE INTERPRETATION OF ORGANIC ANALOGIES IN INSTITUTIONS

Long stay institutions for incapacitated and dependent persons have attracted considerable attention in the literature on care organisations. These institutions seem to present intractable problems in patient care and are prone to periodic scandals. The NHS is no exception and since the mid-sixties, despite improvements in resource allocations (Alaszewski: 1977, Alaszewski: 1978a), there have been a series of scandals in these institutions (Committee of Inquiry: 1969, Committee of Inquiry: 1978).

It is relatively easy to show that these institutions are problematic, but it is more difficult to understand why this should be the case. However, a favourite candidate for blame is the nature of staff attitudes as manifested in staff descriptions of patients.

Most ethnographic studies of long stay institutions indicate that staff use organic analogies such as "vegetables" and "animals" when referring to the patients. Rather than exploring why staff use these analogies, how they may assist them in understanding their situation and in what ways patients are like vegetables, the researchers have argued directly from the statements to actions. It is as though they assumed that if staff refer to patients as animals, then they must also treat them as animals.

This type of argument underlies the following discussion by Brown of the mental hospital as an institution. In it he suggested that animal analogies were an intellectual defence against reality and these analogies were associated with a certain pattern of staff actions, the cruel treatment of patients:

> If those in closest contact with the patient are going to live with some of the things that go on, and keep some kind of self respect they will be helped by the ideas and feelings surrounding such terms as "vegetables", "dozies" and "animals". Such terms immediately open up the way for still greater abuse. Great cruelty is possible in any social situation once persons have in some sense been defined as non-human. (Brown: 1975, p.414)

Towell, in his ethnographic study of a hospital for the mentally ill, was not as cautious as Brown and inextricably mixed statements, ideas (conceptions) and actions. In the following extract Towell discussed the use of vegetable analogies in the psycho-geriatric wards:

> (There was) a tendency for patients to become depersonalised objects of task-centred routines ... In the course of actions patients came to be conceived of as less than fully human ... These conceptions were seen most clearly, however, in terms used to describe patients and a view of their condition as being due to irreversible organic deterioration of the brain ... A student nurse working on the female wards "at the bottom of the ladder" told me "This is a depressing ward. They're vegetables really. All you can do is keep them clean and tidy, and wait for them to die." It was common then to observe the use of terms like "vegetable",

"dregs", "deteriorated" and "demented"
with their dehumanised implications.
(Towell: 1975, p.128)

In Jones's study of mental handicap
hospitals, there was also a close association
between statements, ideas (models) and actions.
Jones distinguished two clusters of ideas and
actions. In the first cluster the staff used a
child model and referred to the patients as
children. She associated a parental role with
this cluster of ideas and actions. On the
"back-wards" researchers recorded a different set
of statements. Jones argued that the behaviour of
patients on these wards made the child model
problematic and it was replaced by an animal model
and the staff referred to the patients as animals.
The associated role was that of zoo keepers.

Particularly sharp responses were found
when the patient's behaviour was of a
particular "dirty" or unpleasant kind.
One male patient who masturbated rectally
was classed as a "filthy" person, and
nurses felt that it was quite legitimate
to beat him, even though such action was
regarded as extreme. (Jones: 1975,
p.109)

Jones argued that certain types of actions,
"beating the patients", were a result of and
legitimated by certain typifications of the
patients. There are two problems in evaluating
this hypothesis. The anecdotal nature of the
evidence makes it difficult to establish how and
in what ways staff models or typifications were
associated with actions. Furthermore, the models
themselves appear to be abstractions created by
the research team from various statements made by
staff in the different hospital studies (Jones:
1975, p.xviii and p.119). This process of
abstraction has decontextualised the models and
may have introduced important distortions. Thus an
important starting point for a study of the
relationship between ideas and action is a more
detailed examination of the ideas.

5.3 ORGANIC TERMS

Discussions by nurses in my study generally

119

did not support the view that references to patients as "children", "animals" or "vegetables" were based on mistaken identity. The statements presented in the first section of Chapter Three clearly used these terms as analogies. However, in some discussions this was not so clear. The following discussions were taken from a written account of the hospital made by a former nurse:

> Whilst I worked in the hospital I became aware of a definite grouping of patients' different abilities. The "higher grade" patients be the majority of them adults were looked upon as children - I worked on Seagull (adult female) ward where at least half of them were elderly yet they were always referred to as "the girls".
> The "low-grade" children, however, were often referred to as if they were no better than animals. I think this assessment was made on their general habits - incontinence - behaviour patterns etc. Attempts to teach this kind of child were usually made in very much the same way as training an animal - habit training/repetition. The multiply handicapped patients were constantly referred to as vegetables. There were often conversations in the "cot-and-chair" wards about euthanasia, wouldn't it be better to let them die, if they were mine etc.

This discussion contained elements of mistaken identity and of analogy. Because it was derived from a written source, it was a commentary on the usage of the terms not an example of usage. It only provided limited information about the context in which the terms were used. However, the discussion also containedthe following analysis of the relationship between these terms and staff actions:

> I think that all three of these descriptions which are often applied are excuses for thinking about the patients in a certain way - if they are like children there is no need to give

them any extra responsibility, if they
are like animals you can treat them as
if they are, as vegetables there is no
need to try to communicate at all. I am
not saying that this is the view either of
all staff or of those who use these
anologies all the time but I do think
that they become a justification for
certain ways of treatment.

In this discussion the terms are clearly seen
as anologies that are used to justify activities
that staff perform for other (unspecified)
reasons, not cases of mistaken identity that cause
certain types of behaviour.

This discussion and the evidence presented in
the first section of Chapter Three utilised the
same terms as Jones identified in her study but in
a different context. In the evidence I have
presented each term was clearly associated with a
category of patients and type of ward. Jones
viewed the "child" model as the dominant model and
argued that it has a certain "elasticity", i.e. it
could be used to cover a certain range of patient
behaviour. When patient behaviour extended beyond
this range, then the model "snapped" and was
replaced by a different model, "patient as animal"
or "patient as filthy person".

Jones tended to argue that when staff
referred to patients as animals or children they
were establishing a direct identity, i.e. patients
were animals, and this caused certain types of
staff behaviour. The respondents, in my study,
argued that these terms were analogies that could
be used to justify different patterns of staff
behaviour.

Some observers have distinguished between the
use of animal terms as analogies and their use to
assert identity. Bettelheim examined one
persistent example of animal terminology applied
to the mentally handicapped - the wild or wolf
children. In this form animal terminology has had
a long association with mental handicap. Wolf or
wild children were children who had been "found"
at the edge of society, in the wilds, and who
exhibited animal-like characteristics when
captured. Both intellectually and socially they
were seen as standing between the social and
natural worlds. Itard's classic study of the Wild
Boy of Aveyron recorded an attempt to socialise

one of those wild children (Malson: 1972).
Pinel, a founding father of modern psychiatry,
referred to the Wild Boy as "an incurable idiot,
inferior to the domestic animal" (Kanner: 1964).
Bettelheim, in his analysis, was concerned to show
that wild children were mentally handicapped
children and their identification as animal was a
mistake. He argued from his own experience that
animal-like behaviour should not be mistaken for
animal identity:

> I can now also see the parallel between
> Singh's story of finding the (wild)
> girls and the wild fantasies we spun
> about the pasts of our autistic
> children when we first meet... (these
> speculations originated) in our
> narcissistic unwillingness to admit
> that these animal-like creatures
> could have had pasts at all similar
> to ours ... Many times when we have
> described the behavior of some of our
> extremely autistic chldren - how they
> urinated and defecated without so much
> as knowing it as they walked or ran
> about; how they could not bear clothes
> but would run about naked; how they
> did not talk but would only scream and
> howl; how they ate only raw food ...
> even persons quite familiar with
> disturbed children would react with
> polite or not so polite disbelief.
> But later, when they met these
> children, their doubts changed to
> complete belief, so that they would
> have been willing to believe almost
> anything told them about the
> children or their pasts.
> On first encounter with their wildness,
> and thereafter, when their total
> withdrawal, their "contrariness", their
> violence, or other types of <u>inhuman,</u>
> <u>animal-like behavior</u> have over-powered
> us and made it harder for us to deal
> rationally with their onslaught, then,
> and despite all our knowledge, we too
> are thrown back for moments to feel they
> are possessed - that <u>they are "animals"</u>.
> (Emphasis is added to the original text)
> (Bettelheim: 1959, pp.456 and 458)

Discussion
      The difference between analogy and identity
underlies Leach's discussion of culture and
communication. Leach was interested in the
process by which "sense images" with which we can
play games in our imagination are related "to
objects and events in the world out-there" (Leach:
1976, p.18). Leach differentiated an index (the
message-bearing entity) from the phenomena it
indicates (the message). He argued that the
relationship could be one of analogy or identity.
In a metonymy, "a part stands for a whole" and the
index "which functions as sign is contiguous to
and part of that which is signified" (Leach: 1976,
p.14). An example of a metonymy is the use of
"the crown" to stand for the monarch. In
metaphorical usage the relationship between the
index and the indicated is non-intrinsic and is
based on asserted similarity. The metaphor is not
part of the indicated, but stands for it by
arbitrary association. One example cited by Leach
was the use of animal analogies.

> But let me go back for a moment to the
> proposition "policemen are pigs". The
> associated is plainly arbitrary and
> therefore symbolic (metaphoric); to
> suppose that it is intrinsic and therefore
> in the nature of a metonymic sign would be
> an error. But, as we shall see, it is an
> important kind of error which all of us
> are inclined to make. It is one of the
> standard devices which we employ to mask
> the fact that nearly everything we say or
> do is full of ambiguity. (Leach: 1976,
> p.21)

      The use of animal analogies in hospitals for
the mentally handicapped appeared to involve this
type of mistake. Metaphor was mistaken for
metonymy by both actors (occasionally) and
observers (frequently). We need to know the
circumstances under which these mistakes are made.
In this chapter, I am more concerned with
understanding more about the animal and organic
terminologies.

5.4 METAPHOR AND METONYMY: PROBLEMS OF MEANING

      In the reported accounts of long stay

institutions, terms such as "animal" tended to be treated as unproblematic descriptions whose meaning was self evident. However, if terms such as "animal" were analogies, not descriptions, then their meaning could no longer be treated as self evident. The next stage of my analysis is to examine the meaning of these terms in the context of the mental handicap hospital.

Since organic analogies have a well established history, one way of unravelling their meaning is to examine historical accounts. One of the earliest accounts was Howe's evidence to the Massachusetts State legislature. This was a seminal account as it formed the basis of subsequent classifications of mental defectives (Howe: 1848). Howe used organic analogies that were organised into a three tier classification. At the lowest level were the "pure idiots", who were referred to as mere organisms.

> Idiots of the lowest class are mere
> organisms, masses of flesh and bone in
> human shape, in which the brain and
> nervous system have no command over the
> system of voluntary muscles; and which
> consequently are without power of
> locomotion, without speech, without any
> manifestation of intellectual or
> affective facilities. (Howe: 1848, p.37)

In the middle were the "fools" who had the power to move and had animal action but were underdeveloped in all other ways.

> Fools are a higher class of idiots, in whom
> the brain and nervous system are so far
> developed as to give partial command
> of the voluntary muscles; who have
> consequently considerable power of
> locomotion and animal action; partial
> development of the affective and
> intellectual facilities, but only the
> faintest glimmer of reason, and very
> imperfect speech. (Howe: 1848, p.37)

At the top were the "simpletons". Although fully developed physically, they were not mentally able and so were not considered socially competent.

> Simpletons are the highest class of idiots,
>   in whom the harmony between the nervous
>   and muscular system is nearly perfect;
>   who consequently have normal powers of
>   locomotion and animal action;
>   considerable activity of the perspective
>   and affective faculties, and reason
>   enough for their simple individual
>   guidance, but not enough for their social
>   relations. (Howe: 1848, p.48)

Three types of development can be identified in this account: physical development; mental development and social or moral development. "Idiots" were not seen as having any development. "Fools" were seen as having physical development. "Simpletons" were seen as having physical and mental development but not social or moral development. The association between moral and social defect is clearly established in Howe's case material. Moral defect was later to become a specific category or class of mental defect. The terms "moral defect" or "moral imbecility" were used as a sub-category of high grade mental defect in the 1913 Mental Deficiency Act. The ability to make moral judgements is seen as an important characteristic of a person in contemporary accounts. For example Voysey (1975: pp.26-36) argued that respondents in her study differentiated between persons and non-persons and that insofar as an individual was not seen as possessing moral character he or she was defined as a non-person.

Howe's account can be summarised diagrammatically where the presence of development is indicated by a plus sign and absence by a minus (Diagram 5.1).

Diagram 5.1   Howe's Classification

	Physical Development	Mental Development	Social/Moral Development
Lowest class	-	-	-
Middle class	+	-	-
Highest class	+	+	-
Normal	+	+	+

Howe's account of the development potential of the different classes shows a great similarity to the accounts of development given by contemporary nurses.

Howe's account exploited certain aspects of Western conceptions of the social and natural universe. Four orders of existence can be isolated from this universe; the adult, the child, the animal and the vegetable. In Howe's account the four orders were arranged in a hierarchy with the independent adult at the peak and the vegetable at the base. Each level built on and shared specific characteristics with the level beneath it but also had its own specific characteristics. Vegetables are alive. Animals add mobility (physical development) to this vegetable existence. Adults add social awareness (social and moral development) to child existence. Looking at these relations in a negative sense and as a process of subtraction then the subtraction of moral sense from the adult state can be seen as creating either a child or high grade subnormal, subtracting both moral sense and mental ability an animal or low grade subnormal and subtracting moral sense, mental ability and physical ability a vegetable or a cot and chair case.

Underlying Howe's account was this process of subtraction. The different levels were the product of different degrees of subtraction. Total subtraction differentiated normality from the lowest level of deficiency:

> those great lazar-houses of London and Paris
> do, sometimes as their records show,
> present such cases of idiocy as, one would
> fain hope, can be found nowhere else. But
> alas! when, overcoming the repugnance to
> close contemplation of utter degradation,
> one looks carefully among the sweepings
> that are cast out by society for something
> that may be saved to humanity, he finds,
> even in our fair commonwealth, breathing
> masses of flesh, fashioned in the shape
> of men, but shorn of all other human
> attributes. (Emphasis in the original
> text) (Howe: 1848, p.37)

The clearest statement of this process of subtraction can be found in Howe's account of the

genesis of idiocy. A moral failure by the parents
was seen as the cause of the loss of one level of
existence during the procreative process. How
else could masturbation cause idiocy? Howe saw
this as a cumulative process in which one level
could be lost in each successive generation
through progressive degeneration and resulting in
the lowest level of idiocy.

> No. 370 ... The causes are probably
> hereditary, he seems to be the last and
> lowest of a constantly degenerating breed.
> The grandparents were intemperate and
> depraved. The children born unto them
> were puny and weak-minded, and they sank
> still lower in the slough of vice and
> depravity. The mother of this boy was
> herself a simpleton; and this was
> her second illegitimate child. Though of
> feeble health, she gave herself up to
> excessive licentiousness, her passions
> becoming almost maniacal. (Howe: 1848,
> p.38)

Discussion

The evidence presented in the second
main section of this Chapter indicates that
organic terms were used metaphorically rather than
metonymically at the Jane Eagle Hospital.

Howe's discussion rested uneasily (and
possible deliberately) on the metaphor/metonymy
interface. It helps us understand the
contemporary use of organic analogies for groups
of patients by making explicit the logic behind
these analogies. In Howe's discussion the
relationship between each class of defective and
the associated organic analogies was not a simple
relationship of either identity or similarity.
They were linked in a more complex way. The
difference between each class of defective was the
same as the difference between the associated
organic terms. Leach has suggested that this is a
common feature of symbolic systems. Symbols are
clustered and interrelated and derive their
meaning from these interrelationships.

> The indices in non-verbal communication
> systems, like the sound elements in
> spoken language, do not have meaning
> as isolates but only as members of sets.

> A sign or symbol only acquires meaning
> when it is discriminated from some other
> contrary sign or symbol. (Leach: 1976,
> p 49)

He gave the following example of meaning created
by context:

> when we dress a bride in a veiled garment
> of white and a widow in a very similar
> veiled garment of black, we are using
> the opposition white/black to express
> not only bride/widow but also good/bad
> as well as a whole range of subsidiary
> harmonic metaphors such as happy/sad,
> pure/contaminated. (Emphasis in the
> original text). (Leach: 1976, p.49)

Leach's analysis developed Levi-Strauss's
earlier work. Organic analogies are not limited
to European cultures. The use of the analogies is
systematically developed in the form of totemism,
a phenomenon widely reported in ethnographies of
other cultures. Levi-Strauss took this phenomenon
as one of his starting points in his analysis of
culture as a mode of communication. He rejected
the Fraserian view that groups were given
names because they were seen as sharing
characteristics with their animal namesakes. In
other words he rejected the view of totemic
categories as metonymic indices of social groups.
Instead he argued that the connection is formal,
logical and metaphorical. The difference between
Animal A and Animal B is the same as the
difference between Group A and Group B. One of the
examples he uses is logically similar to the
examples I have been discussing. It is the Nuer
identification of twins with birds. The main
difference is a logical reversal. In my example
the mentally handicapped are "persons of below"
and the other people are "persons of above". In
the case of Nuer twins the situation is reversed
as follows:

> Twins "are birds", not because they are
> confused with them or because they look
> like them, but because twins, in relation
> to other men, are as "persons of the
> above" to "persons of the below", and, in
> relation to birds, as "birds of the below"

are to "birds of the above". They thus
occupy, as do birds, an intermediary
position between the supreme spirit and
human beings. (Levi-Strauss: 1963,
pp.152-3)

5.5 MEANING AND CONTEXT

Since the meaning of terms is derived from
their context, we can now begin to understand how
Jones developed her version of staff models of the
patients and the mistakes involved. To
recapitulate, Jones argued that the dominant model
of patients, in the mental handicap hospitals
visited by her research team, was the "child
model". She argued that this model had a limited
degree of elasticity and when patient behaviour
went beyond that limit it was replaced by
alternative models, especially patient as animal.
Evidence from the Jane Eagle Hospital
supported Jones's contention that nurses used the
term "child" to refer to all the patients in the
hospital. When staff at the Jane Eagle Hospital
were asked to describe the overall characteristics
of the patients, the term "child" or an equivalent
was used.

Question - How would you describe the
patients in this hospital to someone
who didn't know?

Answer - I'd say that you'd see adults but
remember they're all kids.

Another nurse described these characteristics in
the following way:

Question - Can you describe the hospital?

Answer - It's a home for the mentally
handicapped, Mongols and Spastics.
People with very small heads and people
with very large heads. It's the only
way you can explain. Always remain very
small children. Never older than six
even if they are sixty.

At this level the emphasis was on overall
dependence and lack of intelligence and the term
"child" was used to describe this situation. This

129

association was clear in the following account.

> Question - Could you describe what sort of
> patients the hospital cares for?

> Answer - They cater for young children right
> up to old age.

> Question - What's special about the
> patients?

> Answer - They can't look after themselves.
> They need someone to do it for them.

> Question - Why?

> Answer - Their low intelligence.

Thus at this level the difference between
mentally handicapped people and normal people was
similar to the difference between the children and
adults and this can be represented as follows:

normal : mentally handicapped :: adult : children

However, this was only the first level. In
the discussion of wards a different set of
distinctions was made. For example, the last
interview quoted continued in the following way:

> Question - How would you describe Seagull?

> Answer - Well it's a much higher grade ward,
> much higher grade intelligence. They can
> do a lot more for themselves. You have
> more problems.

Thus within the general class, mentally
handicapped, characterised by dependence and low
intelligence, there were different levels of
dependency and intelligence. The confusion
between the two levels arose because the term
child appeared at both levels.

Level 1 normal : mentally handicapped :: adult :
child

Level 2 high grade : low grade : cot and chair ::
child : animal : vegetable

130

The meaning of the term "child" depended upon its context, the set of terms to which it was contrasted. Thus the meaning of the organic terms was not simply derived from the relationship between the term and a class of patients but was related to the differences between different organic terms and the ways in which these differences were associated with classes of patients. Indeed respondents found no difficulty in referring to high grade patients both as children and as adults. The former term was used when respondents wanted to stress the limitations of high grade patients when contrasted with ordinary adults, the latter was used when respondents wanted to stress the superior abilities and potential of high grade patients.

We can now begin to understand why researchers have mistaken a metaphorical usage for a metonymic one. The meaning of terms such as child is dependent on the context (and purpose) of their use. Researchers have decontextualised this usage. Bourdieu describes this in the following way:

> (The) plurality of meanings (of symbols and words) at once different and more or less closely interrelated is a product of scientific collection. Each of the significations collected exists in its practical state only in the relationship between a scheme (or the product of a scheme, a word for example) and a specific situation. (Bourdieu: 1977, pp.122-3)

The process of decontextualisation has been common in studies by social anthropologists of the symbolic systems (ritual, myth, totemism etc.) of other cultures. Goody pointed out that the techniques anthropologists use to study these symbolic systems have seriously distorted these systems by decontextualising them. Anthropologists have recorded oral traditions, myths, classifications etc. in written form, frequently in graphs or tables. These written forms have tended to remove the symbols from their context and have destroyed the essential ambiguity, the context specific nature, of the symbols.

What I have suggested here is that this

> standardisation, especially as epitomised in the Table consisting of $\underline{k}$ columns and $\underline{r}$ rows, is essentially the result of applying graphic techniques to oral material. The result is often to freeze a contextual statement into a system of permanent oppositions, an outcome that may simplify reality for the observer but often at the expense of a real understanding of the actor's frame of reference. (Goody: 1977, pp.71-3)

Goody's comments can be applied to the analysis of researchers such as Jones because Jones provided little information on the different contexts and meanings of the terms she recorded. However, Goody's comments could also be read as a criticism of the analytical procedures I have adopted in this chapter. Although I have treated terms such as "child" as context specific, I have treated one particular relationship as the dominant one, "high grade" as "child", "low grade" as "animal" and "cot and chair patient" as "vegetable". I have treated this one as the dominant one because it is related to clear historical antecedents.

There is an essential difference between the classifications studied in this book and those studied by anthropologists. In anthropological analysis the problems are created by the imposition of a literate form, the graph or table, on an open fluid oral form. In the mental handicap hospital, I was recording talk but this talk was based on a written form with an institutionalised model of transmission (nurse training), and clear links could be established between written records and current talk. Thus my analysis was not so much an imposition of a structure as a rediscovery of an implicit structure on which current talk was based. However, it is important to remember that this structure did not represent some rigid set of constraints but was used and manipulated by contemporary actors to get things done.

Goody's analysis provides a means for understanding the relationship between contemporary talk about the patients and historical accounts. In non-literate societies records are memorised. Each act of reproduction of this record also tends to be a productive or

innovative act. New elements are constantly
incorporated into the records but in a fairly
anonymous fashion.

> In oral societies a man's achievement, be it
> ballad or shrine, tends to get
> incorporated (or rejected) in an anonymous
> fashion. It is not that the creative
> element is absent, though its character is
> different. And it is not that a mysterious
> collective authorship, closely in touch
> with the collective consciousness, does
> what individuals do in literate cultures.
> It is rather that the individual signature
> is always getting rubbed out in the
> process of generative transmission.
> (Goody: 1977, p.27)

In oral societies knowledge is produced and
reproduced in the same act and this act rapidly
becomes anonymous. Memories are short. Status
accrues to the reproducer (who is also an
innovator and producer). In literate societies
the production and reproduction of knowledge are
clearly separated and status accrues to the
producer rather than the reproducer. Production
of knowledge is discontinuous, personalised and
fixed in the literate form. The form of
reproduction can vary but is often continuous,
anonymous and oral. In this chapter, I have been
looking at the personalised production of
knowledge, i.e. the Howe report, whereas the
interview material was derived from the anonymous
acts of the reproduction of this knowledge.

5.6   CONCLUSION AND DISCUSSION

In this chapter, I have developed my analysis
of the ward system by examining the analogies
associated with different classes of patients. I
have argued that previous researchers have tended
to misunderstand the meaning and usage of terms
such as child and animal. These researchers have
mistaken metaphor for metonymy and have
substituted literal for figurative meanings. The
decontextualisation of the usage has limited a
fuller examination of meaning. I have argued that
when nurses referred to low grades as "animals"
and cot and chair patients as "vegetables" they
are establishing an equivalence between the

differences between low grade patients/cot and chair patients and the differences between animals and vegetables, i.e. the absence of mobility. In contrasting low grade patients and high grade patients a different set of contrasts could be used, i.e. "child" to "adult", emphasising the greater social skills of high grade patients.

The failure to differentiate between metaphor and metonymy is related to the decontextualisation of usage. Jones did not examine the way in which the term "child" was used in different contexts and the differences of meaning it had in these contexts. As a result she argued that the meaning of the term was fixed and when this meaning could no longer be imposed on the situation the term child had to be replaced with another one.

I have not in this chapter dealt with the second aspect of the argument, viz. terms such as animal not only describe the patients they also prescribe certain types of relationships. If the patients are referred to as animals then do nurses themselves act as zoo keepers physically controlling the patients and do doctors act as vets? The relationship between ideas and actions forms the main theme of Part Three of this book, Chapters Six to Eight. In this concluding section I shall make some preliminary comments.

I have in this part of the book concentrated on the meaning of the different classifications of patients, i.e. examined the information they contain. In Part Three I shall examine the function, i.e. what the classifications do. The separation between meaning and functions, between understanding and doing, is only an analytic device and analysis of the meaning has already cast some light on function. Broadly two alternative interpretations can be made of the functions of patient classification:

1. they describe a certain kind of reality and prescribe appropriate actions;

2. they are used by the staff to justify and legitimate actions whose origins can be found in the practical situation.

The first interpretation would give primacy to the ideas and would see them as a set of rules that the staff follow.

The first type of interpretation is implicit in the work of Schutz. Schutz argued that the process of classifying and naming is the basis of human actions.

> the outer world is not experienced as an
> arrangement of individual unique objects,
> disposed in space and time, but as
> "mountains", "trees", "animals",
> "fellow-men". (Schutz: 1971, pp.7-8)

These names carry with them information and expectations, especially information about the behaviour of the named objects and of other actors. As long as the object or situation conforms sufficiently to previous equivalent objects of situations, the name effectively acts as a rule for behaviour. This is clear in the following example given by Schutz.

> I take it for granted that my action
> (say putting a stamped and duly addressed
> envelope in a mailbox) will induce
> anonymous fellow-men (postmen) to perform
> typical actions (handling the mail) in
> accordance with typical in-order-to
> motives (to live up to their occupational
> duties) with the result that the state
> affairs projected by me (delivery of the
> letter to the addressee within reasonable
> time) will be achieved. (Schutz; 1971,
> p.25)

I was tempted to interpret the classification of patients at the Jane Eagle hospital as a set of rules for dealing with the patients. For example the ward level classification appeared to provide information about the type of routine appropriate for the different grades of patient. Indeed for a time I did interpret the grade classification in this way. However, evidence already presented and to be presented in Part Three indicated that staff did not treat the grade system as a set of rules. They manipulated it. For example they used the low grade wards as refractory wards for difficult high grade patients. As the nurse in Section One of this chapter said, nurses used descriptions as "excuses for thinking about the patients in certain ways".
Bourdieu has criticised the conceptualisation

of a culture as a series of rules and has emphasised the importance of individual choice and strategy. The ability of the individual to exploit depends on the ambiguity of most social situations:

> the fact remains that the differences
> between the two parties are never
> clear-cut, so that each can play as
> the ambiguities and equivocations which
> this indeterminacy lends to conduct.
> (Bourdieu: 1977, p.14)

Bourdieu suggested that the importance of rules lies not in the way in which they cause behaviour but rather in the way in which they justify and legitimate behaviour. The egotistic, self interested behaviour of the individual is reinterpreted as rule based and group oriented behaviour.

> strategies directly oriented towards the
> primary profit of practice (e.g. the
> prestige accruing from a marriage) are
> almost always accompanied by second-order
> strategies whose purpose is to give
> apparent satisfaction to the demands of
> the official rule, and thus to compound
> the satisfactions of enlightened self
> interest with the advantage of ethical
> impeccability.(Bourdieu: 1977, p.22)

In the third part of this book, I shall consider three aspects of the relationship between ideas and actions. In Chapter Six I shall examine the ways in which the structure of ideas was maintained through the pattern of nurse training. In Chapter Seven I shall consider the relationship between the ward classification and the provision of basic care in the hospital. In Chapter Eight I shall consider the practical strategies adopted for the care and control of three "high grade" patients.

CHAPTER 6
THE WARD   SYSTEM AS A SOURCE   OF KNOWLEDGE: NURSE
TRAINING

6.1   INTRODUCTION (This   chapter is   adapted from
Alaszewski: 1977)

The   ward classification   of   patients had   a
visible   form   in   the   layout of   villas   in   the
hospital, but the significance and meaning of this
layout would   not be   obvious to an   outsider.   To
understand the   significance of this   structure an
outsider had   to be   taught and had to be socialised
into the   hospital   culture.   Although the hospital
was staffed by a   number of different occupational
groups,   such   as   doctors,   physiotherapists,
occupational   therapists,   and ancillary   workers,
the   largest   group with   the most   patient contact
was   the nurses.   Therefore nurses   played a   key
part in   maintaining the   culture of   the hospital
and   in socialising   new members   of   the hospital
staff.   In   this   chapter I   shall   discuss   the
process of   nurse socialisation   as it   related to
the classification of patients in the hospital and
strategies of patient management in the hospital.

6.2   THE FORMAL ORGANISATION OF NURSE TRAINING

At the   time of   my research   nurse education
was   based   on   an   apprenticeship type   training
and the staffing requirements of the hospital were
given   precedence over   the educational   needs of
nurses   (Towell: 1975).   The   regulations   for
clinical   experience, set   by the   General Nursing
Council   for England   and   Wales   (GNC), were   the
major   means of   maintaining   the balance   between
educational   and   service   needs.   The   Briggs
Committee   had   reported   and   its   proposals   for
changing nurse training structure were accepted in

principle by the DHSS in 1976 (DHSS: 1976) but little change had occurred in the pattern of training at ward level. The regulations for clinical experience formed an important part of the system of nurse training. These regulations had to be interpreted by the Senior Nursing Officer responsible for allocating nurses to wards. The way, in which they were interpreted, related to the internal structure of wards in the hospital and played an important role in the socialisation of nurses.

Nurse training at the Jane Eagle Hospital was made up of two separate and sometimes unrelated parts, short periods of formal instruction by tutors in a nurse training school and longer periods of informal instruction by trained nurses and other specialists in the working environment. To ensure that nurses obtain "adequate" experience the GNC stipulate that during their training nurses had to spend certain minimum periods either with specified types of patients or in specific working situations or environments. The GNC regulations were broadly phrased and gave a large area of discretion to nursing administrators, as shown in Table 6.1.

Table 6.1 Summary of GNC regulations for practical instruction for the mental subnormality register (specified periods given in weeks)

Ward Experience

Newly admitted patients	12
Subnormal and/or severely subnormal adults	12
Subnormal and/or severely subnormal children	12
Physically handicapped or physically sick pts.	12

Other Ward Experience
Nights	12-36

Therapy Environments
School training methods	12
Occupational and/or industrial therapy	12

Other Training Situations
Local authority (optional)	4-12

Total (min. to max)	88-120
Total length of course	156

Nurse Training

The GNC regulations for the training of nurses for the mental subnormality register have been derived from the regulations for nurses training for the general register. Table 6.2 shows the similarity in structure between conditions of approval of training schools for the general register and the mental subnormality register

Table 6.2 <u>Conditions of approval of training schools</u> (types of clinical experience which must be available)

<u>General register</u>

General medical nursing of men and women

General surgical nursing of men and women, including gynaecological and genito-urinary nursing

Operating Theatre

Accident/Casualty and/or Out-Patient Clinics

Ear, nose and throat, ophthalmic and orthopaedic conditions (either in the wards or in out-patients clinics)

One or more specialty

<u>Register for nurses of the mentally subnormal</u>

Nursing care of subnormal and severely subnormal children and adults

Nursing care of sick and physically handicapped patients

Experience in school training methods and occupational, social and recreational therapy

In general hospitals, wards are grouped according to function and on each type of ward a nurse is expected to learn a specialised skill. In the general hospital, it is self evident that a nurse cannot be considered trained until he or she has worked on all types of wards and acquired the whole range of basic skills. Even in general hospitals, the system of allocation of training nurses to wards has been criticised because it can create an excessive amount of instability and can prevent the creation of nurse-patient relations. Menzies (1960) argued that instability and the lack of stablility in nurse-patient relationships were not the unfortunate side effect of the training programme, but were its unconscious objective. She saw rapid staff movement as a social defence mechanism intended to allay anxiety by preventing excessive involvement by the nurses in the lives of individual patients.

The GNC regulations for the mental subnormality register did not have the same self evident characteristic as the equivalent regulations for the general register. The GNC regulations did not conform to the internal organisation of the Jane Eagle hospital. For example, the GNC regulations specified that nurses training for the register must have twelve weeks' experience of working with newly admitted patients. At the Jane Eagle Hospital there was no special ward for these patients. Newly admitted patients were not at any time differentiated or separated from other patients. The GNC regulations did not have any meaning in this context.

Given the broad framework of the GNC regulations, especially for the mental subnormality register, there was considerable discretion left to individual hospitals in allocating nurses to wards and other training environments. Therefore the principles adopted by individual hospitals were very important. At the Jane Eagle Hospital, the Senior Nursing Officer was responsible for the allocation of training nurses. He adopted a principle based on a regular rotation of training nurses so that, as far as possible all training nurses during their training worked on all wards. Training nurses were allocated to wards for 8-12 week periods and then moved. The Senior Nursing Officer was "playing safe" and ensuring that training nurses had a "wider" range of experience than that stipulated by the GNC. The result of this policy, from the point of view of the training nurse, was constant movement between different wards, and, from the point of view of other staff and patients on the ward, was a constant stream of new student nurses. In the next section I examine the evidence from the ward point of view.

6.3 ALLOCATION OF NURSES TO WARDS: THE CREATION
OF AN UNSTABLE ENVIRONMENT OF CONSTANT CHANGES

The ward environment could be characterised
as one in which a relatively stable group of
patients was cared for by a constantly changing
group of nurses. On the 1st March 1974,
Ravensbourn Ward, a ward with 28 profoundly and
multiply handicapped patients, had an
establishment of 13 nurses on day duty. However,
during the next six months of 1974 nearly three
times that number of nurses (37) worked as
"permanent" staff on the ward. Of the 13 nurses
who were allocated as permanent staff to the ward
at the start of the period, only 4 were still
working on the ward after six months. In addition
to the 37 "permanent nurses", 47 nurses worked
temporarily on the ward during this period.

I recorded the number of nurses who worked
during a 76 week period on Seagull Ward, a ward
with approximately 30 mildly handicapped women
patients. The ward had an overall establishment
of 8 nurses. 42 nurses worked as permanent staff
on the ward. 81 nurses worked as temporary staff
on the ward and worked 11% of the 2,520 nurse
shifts worked during this period.

The "permanent" nurses worked on the ward for
an average of 14.5 weeks but there was a wide
variation in the length of time "permanent" staff
worked on the ward (See Table 6.3). Half the
permanent staff worked less than 10 weeks whereas
two nurses worked 38 weeks or more, though no
nurse worked the full 76 weeks.

If the figures are examined in terms of
category of nurse, night staff and trained,
training and untrained day staff, then it is
possible to identify the effect of student
allocation policy. Trained staff and night staff
stayed on the ward longer than training and
untrained staff. 7 night staff worked on average
19.6 weeks each. 12 trained day staff worked on
average 22.3 weeks each, nearly twice as long as
the 11 training staff who worked on average 10.5
weeks, and the 12 untrained staff who worked on
average 12.2 weeks. Furthermore, of the five
"established" nurses on the ward, i.e. nurses who
worked more than 38 weeks out of 76 weeks on the
ward, two were night nurses, two were trained

Table 6.3 <u>Distribution of length of time worked by permanent staff allocated to Seagull Ward during a 76 week period</u> (mean = 14.5 weeks)

<u>Weeks worked</u>	<u>Number of nurses</u>
0-5	11
6-10	10
11-15	5
16-20	3
21-25	2
26-30	3
31-35	2
over 36	6

staff and only one was from the other categories, a nursing assistant.

Although the average length of time that untrained and training nurses worked on the ward was similar, the distribution of the length of time for which these two categories of nurses were allocated to the ward was different (See Table 6.4).

Table 6.4 <u>Distribution of length of time worked by untrained nurses and training nurses allocated as permanent day staff to Seagull Ward during a 76 week period</u>

<u>Weeks worked</u>	<u>Untrained</u>	<u>Trained</u>
0-10	9	6
11-20	1	4
over 21	2	1

Untrained nurses either worked for a short period on the ward (9 out of 12 nurses), or else worked longer periods (2 out of 12 nurses) and became "established" on the ward. Only one untrained nurse fell in the middle group. On the other hand, a substantial minority of nurses in training fell in this middle group (4 out of 11 nurses) and the majority worked for up to 10 weeks (6 out of 11 nurses). These figures were the result of the policy adopted by the nursing officer that nurses in training should move every 8-12 weeks. Only one nurse in training worked longer than 20 weeks and her case was exceptional. She first worked as a nursing assistant on the ward for 10 weeks and, after her initial 6 week course in nurse training school, her first placement was on Seagull Ward where she worked a further 19 weeks.

6.4 NURSE MOVEMENT AND WARD ORGANISATION

The effects of these various nurse movements were to create an environment of instability for the patients. Only 5 out of the 8 staff needed to provide a minimum "cover" for Seagull Ward stayed on the ward for even half of the 76 week period. Two of these were night nurses, who had limited contact with the patients and the other two (ward sister and charge nurse) had administrative duties that reduced the length of time they could spend with the patients. This meant that the responsibility for maintaining ward "culture", i.e. the standards and pattern of care, and teaching it to new ward nurses, tended to be passed to the remaining established nurse, an untrained nursing assistant. The majority of patient care was carried out by a group of constantly changing training and untrained nurses supervised by the three established day staff.

These observations are not new. King, Raynes and Tizard (1971) made similar observations:

> As a group, the hospital wards are likely
> to have thirteen times as many new
> staff working in them over a
> 6-month period as the hostels and
> six times as many as the voluntary
> homes. Continuity in child care is
> clearly more likely to be found in
> the hostels and the voluntary homes than
> it is in the hospitals, where children
> are likely to be cared for by, on average,
> more than twenty new members of
> staff during a period of 6 months.

However, King, Raynes and Tizard did not use

staff mobility as an independent variable. They argued that the degree of staff mobility was dependent on the orientation (child or institution) of the unit. Therefore, they did not offer any suggestions for reducing mobility and did not make any predictions about the effects of reduced staff mobility.

Some researchers believe that the constant movement of nursing staff is related to and even responsible for many of the negative features of patient care they have observed , especially rigid routines and depersonalised block treatment of patients (Menzies: 1960). Associated with these were negative features of ward organisation, especially the lack of ward teams and the existence of rigidly defined roles. The negative features of patient care and ward organisation were related to each other and were both the product of the same phenomenon - the need for rapid socialisation of new nurses because of the constant turnover of nurses.

Rigid routines of basic care activities, block treatment of patients and rigid classifications of patients were part of a pattern of adjustment to a high staff turnover. All wards in the hospital had a similar rigid routine or pattern of care activities. This meant that once nurses had learnt the routine in one ward, they could, with minimal adjustments, work on all similar wards in the hospital. Block and group treatment of patients resulted from the interaction between the routine and a classification of patients. The care patients received was related to the ward routine which in turn was related to their classification, both within the hospital and on the ward. This meant that a nurse on a new ward learnt how a particular patient was affected by the ward routine by learning how the patient was classified by other nurses on the ward. This information told the nurse what "sort" of patient he or she was dealing with and therefore rather than learning about the patients as individuals and learning how to establish relationships with individuals, albeit handicapped individuals, the new nurse was learning about patients' group affiliations and how to manage groups of patients.

The high turnover of nursing staff on wards also accounted for the lack of stable ward teams, despite the high value placed on teamwork by nursing administrators and the dominant place of teams, ward teams and multi-disciplinary teams. The nursing administrators frequently referred to the importance of developing ward teams. However the constant movement of nurses prevented the emergence of real teams. Strauss et al (1964) have argued that movement is disruptive to order. They included routine as one of the positive aspects of order. They, meant negotiated or flexible routine arising out of the situation, rather than the rigid routine of basic care activities evident in the Jane Eagle Hospital. Movement was disruptive to flexible routines and they had to be continually reformed or replaced by rigid centralised routines.

> The perennial transfer of nurses from
> one ward to another and from one shift
> to another allows some nurses to discover
> genuine satisfactions in working at the
> hospital; but this transfer system can
> also be immensely disrupting to nurses
> who have nicely managed their
> environments. Transfer not merely
> shatters routine and necessitates the
> learning of new routines, but it also
> means that new alliances must be made,
> new channels of negotiations found,
> new conditions of work be handled. To
> some degree at least a new environment
> must be managed (Strauss et al: 1964).

The ability of nursing administrators to maintain the myth of ward teams in the face of the evidence of constant change in the wards was related to the ambiguity of the term "ward team". The definition of "team" used here is derived from the work of the Tavistock, especially the analysis by Trist (Trist et al: 1963) of work groups at the coal face. They defined the conditions in which teams could develop as those in which a stable group of individuals coped with a specified task requiring the utilisation of specialised skills by individual members.

A team emerged when the required division of labour was produced by internal negotiations within the group. Each individual accepted responsibility for the achievement of the common group goal and utilised his or her skills in the best possible fashion for the achievement of this goal. They contrasted this with the situation in which a division of labour was imposed on a group, a task was fragmented into a number of parts and each individual was concerned only with the accomplishment of his or her part without achievement of the total goal.

A precondition for the development of teams which act cohesively is an established and relatively stable membership because, only where there is established staff can stable relations between staff members and flexible patterns of work with informal specialisation, develop. This does not mean that a stable group of staff will inevitably form a team, but that stability is a necessary although not sufficient condition. Instability produces the opposite to a team, a group of staff rigidly divided into fixed and defined roles. In an unstable, changing situation individuals must be interchangeable so that any one role can be performed by a wide range of individuals. This interchangeability is created by a rigid division of labour in which different care and therapy tasks are allocated to roles rather than individuals. At the Jane Eagle Hospital the policy of constantly moving nurses between wards meant that the ward team was part of the official rhetoric of senior managers rather than a reality of ward organisation.

6.5 NURSING SUBCULTURE AND THE EXPERIENCED NURSE

Nurses at the Jane Eagle Hospital, especially on the wards, had adjusted to change. In their subculture a virtue has been made out of necessity. Nurses on ·the wards saw staff movements as inevitable, because of recurrent staffing crisis, and argued that it was therefore an advantage for nurses to be moved regularly so that they could get a wide experience of the hospital and be ready to work on any ward in a crisis. This recognition of the inevitable can be seen in the following statement made by a recently qualified staff nurse:

> Student nurses should be moved regularly
> because then they know all the patients
> in the hospital. This means that if they
> have to be shifted they will know the
> patients on the ward on which they worked.

> I know all the patients in the hospital
> except the Pelican and the Hawk patients
> and this means I can work on any ward on
> which I am put.

The emphasis on knowing all the patients and
being able to work on any ward in the hospital
meant that experience gained from constant
movement between the wards and informal
instruction on the wards was more highly valued
than knowledge gained by formal instruction in
nurse training school.

> I often felt that the school training lacked
> relevance to what we had to deal with
> on the wards. The emphasis of the
> teaching in school was on clinical types,
> illness, anatomy and physiology, nursing
> procedures. The work on the ward apart
> from basic nursing care was mainly to be
> with the patients - talking, cuddling,
> helping them to develop skills.
> The knowledge acquired on the wards was
> far more relevant and useful. The
> experiences gained from working on
> the wards are how you learn to deal with
> the patients.

Experience acquired an almost mystical
property, as something a person acquired after
long periods of working with many different types
of patients. This can be seen in the following
statement made by a ward charge nurse with long
service in mental handicap hospitals:

> I've been in nursing 21 years so I've learnt
> what the patients are like. It's really
> a matter of experience and getting to know
> your patients. This is difficult to
> explain to someone who has only just
> started.

A statement from the preliminary report of a
research project at another mental handicap
hospital indicates the same set of ideas:

> Staff with several years' experience
> of working in the hospital are likely to
> have worked in most if not all parts of
> it. As many have trained there, this

147

> common background of experience may
> explain the apparent homogeneity. Staff
> are expected to be able to work in any
> part of the hospital ... They are all
> Balderton nurses. It is almost as if
> there is an ideal of a Balderton nurse
> as a "well-rounded personality", able to
> cope almost indiscriminately with the
> needs of the widely varying categories of
> patients, however these categories be
> defined within the hospital.
> (Dartington et al: 1973)

There was a systematic ambiguity in nurses'
usage of the term "experience". The term
experience was used both to describe the process
of becoming an experienced nurse and the result of
this process, the quality of experience that
differentiated the experienced from the
inexperienced nurse. This ambiguity created a
confusion between the process and the end product
so that the acquisition of experience tended to be
seen as an automatic process that resulted from
the continual movement of nurses between wards. To
avoid this confusion the term experience can be
used to describe the process and the term
competence to describe the quality.

Differentiating between the process,
experience, and the product, competence, makes it
possible to identify a small group of nurses who
were experienced, but incompetent. In other words
they had the same experience as other nurses, but
were not treated as competent. These individuals
were differentiated from competent nurses by three
criteria: (1) they were socially isolated and not
regarded as part of the hospital's community of
nurses and participants in the hospital nursing
subculture, (2) their formal qualifications were
treated as paper qualifications resulting from
book knowledge and (3) it was believed that they
were unable to manage the patients and were
therefore seen as a liability to other staff,
especially on ambulant wards.

It was this latter criterion, ability to
manage or control patients, that provided a clue
to the nature of experience and competence.
Competence was the practical ability to manage and
care for a group or ward of patients on a day to
day basis. Experience was not learning how to
establish relationships with individual patients,

148

but learning how to divide patients on a ward into
groups or categories and learning how to manage
these different groups. It was not learning about
individuals and their personalities, it was
learning classifications and patient management
strategies.

6.6 SKILLS AND WARD CLASSIFICATIONS

Although nurses at the Jane Eagle Hospital
could be differentiated in terms of their
experience and competence and were expected to
work on different types of ward, it was also
accepted that different sorts of nurse were suited
for different types of ward. Nurses, who were good
on cot and chair wards, might not be so good on
high grade wards. Nurses were seen as having
different personalities and social backgrounds.
The Charge Nurse on Seagull (high grade) ward
assessed this in the following way:

A person who is great on Ravensbourn
and Beaver, someone like Denise
Donnison,can be useless on here.

Question - What do you think makes a good
nurse on Seagull?

Answer - Denise Donnison does not
seem to develop that inter-personal
relationship with the patients. She
develops a relationship. She tries very
hard to but she sees it as part of
"the job".

Question - Too clinical?

Answer - Its a natural thing. The
likes of Judy, Nina, and Tessa they spend
hours with a patient just talking to them,
doing things with them. Tessa would do the
bathing and it would take her from 6 to
8. You'd go down to see what she was
doing. She'd spend hours with the lowest
grade patient... People like Kirstie, she
didn't quite have that. She could clean my
lockers out, sort all the clothes, re-mark
all the lockers, take the patients out for
a walk but she didn't quite have that.

The type of skill and personality required was generally seen as varying with the grade of patient. One experienced nurse described the relationship in the following way:

> Seagull (high grade) is a ward for female ambulant patients who can communicate quite well and who can do most things for themselves. There are many kinds of behaviour problems and it takes a mature and insightful person to deal with them - calm and kind but firm.

> Pelican Ward (low grade) is for adult females who are ambulant but have very little speech. They need help with dressing, feeding and many are doubly incontinent. As they are adult sized but with very little ability to communicate, much of their frustration comes out in aggression. Nursing them requires confidence, firmness, kindness and stamina as the physical workload can be great and it is combined with the mental stress.

> Ravensbourn (cot and chair) is a ward for multiply handicapped people. Their physical and mental handicaps are so severe that it is sometimes difficult to communicate with them at all. These people need physical care, encouragement to develop any possible skills and warmth and affection. Nurses must enjoy physical contact and be prepared to see any minute improvement as the major achievement it is. Kindness and patience are essential.

6.7 CONCLUSION

If the classification of ward patients was a special source of knowledge then its maintenance depended on the existence of a system for reproducing this knowledge. The system of allocating nurses to wards played an essential role in socialising new nurses and in reproducing the knowledge base of the hospital. As the new nurses were moved regularly between the wards they found it difficult to develop relationships with individual patients and therefore it was difficult for new nurses to get to know the patients as people. Instead they learnt to view patients as members of classes or grades and learnt methods of managing patients as groups.

The experience gained through constant movement between wards created the competent nurse. This nurse had the skill and ability to work on any ward in the hospital. The patients on different types of ward were seen as having different needs and presenting different management problems and different types of nurse were seen as suited to different types of ward.

CHAPTER 7
MEALTIMES: VARIATIONS IN ACTIVITY PATTERNS BETWEEN
WARDS

7.1 INTRODUCTION

Until recently social researchers have tended
to neglect the analysis of everyday life in
advanced capitalist society. Social
anthropologists have, in their concern with the
total life of small groups, devoted a lot of
attention to both the dramatic and mundane
dimensions of everyday life in other cultures.
These often seem strange and exotic to social
anthropologists and therefore interesting in their
own right. In contrast everyday life in western
society seems mundane. The privacy of domestic
life in our society has reinforced the problems of
research.
Research in institutions is an exception. In
these organisations, activities such as eating,
disposing of bodily waste and sleeping, form an
important focus of organisational activity. In
this chapter, I examine one of these activities -
eating. I shall examine the way in which these
activities were organised on three different
wards, Seagull, a high grade ward, Pelican, a low
grade ward and Ravensbourn, a cot and chair ward.
I shall examine the ways in which the structure of
ward classification related to the patterns of
social action in the institution.

7.2 THE MEANING OF MEALS

At the Jane Eagle Hospital, both staff and
patient activities were dominated by the provision
of the basic necessities of life. In the hospital
basic care activities were organised into a
routine. The routine was made of a number of

152

different activities, including sleeping/waking, dressing/undressing, eating/drinking, disposing of bodily waste, and maintaining personal hygiene. Just as basic care activities were central to hospital life, so mealtimes were central to basic care activities. The other activities tended to cluster around the mealtime and mealtimes formed "the major periods of daily life" (Bury: 1974, p.249).

The main function of basic care activities was to satisfy the physical and biological needs of the patient. However this was not their only function (or the main reason for their theoretical interest to me). Anthropological studies suggest that activities such as eating not only do something, satisfy hunger, but can also say something. Meals can be treated as a code that contains a message. If food may be considered as a code, what sort of message is it encoding? Douglas has suggested meals encode messages about social relations.

> If food is treated as a code, the messages
> it encodes will be found in the pattern of
> social relations being expressed. The
> message is about different degrees of
> hierarchy, inclusion and exclusion,
> boundaries and transactions across the
> boundaries. Like sex, the taking of food
> has a social component, as well as a
> biological one. Food categories therefore
> encode social events. (Douglas: 1975,
> p.249)

In the mental handicap hospital, the messages were about the social relations between the patients and the hospital staff.

How can the "message" of a meal be deciphered? Douglas started with Levi-Strauss's work on table manners and food categories (Levi-Strauss: 1970). However as she pointed out, Levi-Strauss's analysis is not much use to the empirical researcher because "he is looking for a precoded, panhuman message in the language of food", and is therefore not really interested in "the small-scale social relations which generate the codifications and are sustained by it" (Douglas: 1975, p.250). Douglas suggested that a meal can be read in the same way as a sentence. Meaning is created by both the sequence of elements in a meal (syntagm) and the alternative set of elements that could be substituted at a given point in the chain (paradigm). Drawing on the work of the linguist Halliday (1961), Douglas showed how the elements of meals can be compared to linguistic units. Just as an individual sentence has a structure of grammatical relationships and lexical items so an individual meal can be broken into constituent parts, e.g. cheese, and grammatical relations, e.g. first course.

Douglas argued that the meaning of any particular meal, e.g. a Christmas dinner, can be found in the relationship between the structure of that meal and other meals. The internal structure of meals is related to their external relationships. Douglas argued that domestic or family meals are ordered in scale of importance and grandeur through the week and the year. Meals on special occasions are more elaborate versions of simple everyday meals. But all meals possess the same internal structure and can be judged by the same "grammatical rules". Therefore each individual meal can be assessed in the context of other meals.

> The smallest, meanest meal metonymically
> figures the structure of the grandest,
> and each unit of the grand meal figures
> again the whole meal - or the meanest
> meal. The perspective created by these
> repetitive analogies invests the
> individual meal with additional meaning.
> Here we have the principle we were
> seeking, the intensifier of meaning, the
> selection principle. A meal stays in the
> category of meal only in so far as it
> carries this structure which allows the
> part to recall the whole. Hence the
> outcry against allowing the sequence of
> soup and pudding to be called a meal.
> (Douglas: 1975, pp.257-8)

Douglas argued that English meals have a recognisable structure and common pattern. Douglas argued that there were a number of separable levels or in her terms "units" to this pattern. For example an individual meal could be considered in relation to the other meals in a day, or in terms of the relationship of courses within it. Douglas distinguishes five main levels or types of units.

* Daily Menu
* Meal
* Course
* Helping
* Mouthful

She argued that each unit has its own structure of elements. Different social groups will have different daily menus but, in England, these will follow a recognisable pattern. She suggested that the daily menu in England is made up of four distinctive types of meal, an early meal, a main meal, a light meal and a snack. Different social groups will organise these elements in different ways and give them different names. Douglas (1975: pp.251-2) provides the following structure for the English menu.

<u>Unit: Daily Menu</u>

Elements of the Primary Structure   E, M, L, S
                         (early, main, light, snack)

Primary stuctures	EML EMLS (conflated as EML (S))
Exponents of these elements (primary classes of unit "meal")	E : 1 (breakfast) M : 2 (dinner) L : 3 S : 4
Secondary structures	ELaSaM ELaM EMLbSb EMSaLc
Exponents of secondary elements (systems of secondary classes of unit "meal")	La : 3.1 (lunch) Lb : 3.2 (high tea) Lc : 3.3 (supper) Sa : 4.1 (afternoon tea) Sb : 4.2 (nightcap)
Systems of sub-classes of unit "meal"	E : 1.1 (English breakfast) 1.2 (Continental breakfast)

At the next level, the meal unit, Douglas provided a similar example of the potential structure of the main meal. She suggested that main meals are made up of courses, e.g. main

155

course, but they may vary in the number of courses. All have a main course and a sweet but in addition they may have a first course such as soup or antipasto.

Unit : Meal, Class : Dinner

Elements of primary   F,S,M,W,Z ("first", "second", "main", "sweet", "savoury")

Primary structure   MW, MWZ, MZW, FMW, FMWZ, FMZW, FSMW, FSMWZ, FSMZW (conflated as F(S) MW(Z))

Exponents of these
        elements   F : 1 (antipasto)
(primary classes of   S : 2 (fish)
  unit courses)   M : 3 (entree)
                          W : 4 (dessert)
                          Z : 5 (cheese)

These patterns could be identified in the hospital. The daily menu was relatively simple. Each ward had a breakfast, a main meal and a tea (EMLb) and on ambulant wards there was a late snack (Sb). Each meal was simple. For example the main meal was a main course followed by a dessert (MW). For patients eating minced diet (mainly on cot and chair wards) the first and second courses were differentiated only in flavour not in terms of the other contrasts such as hot and cold, bland and spiced, liquid and semi-liquid (Douglas: 1975, p.255). The six difficult feeders on one low grade ward had scrambled egg, porridge and bread mixed together for their breakfast. Even the non-minced meals were criticised for their lack of structure. One nurse described them in the following way:

> The meals are unbalanced. They think
> nothing of serving stodge, followed by
> stodge, pastry followed by pastry.

This nurse was arguing that hospitals' meals were not proper meals. The elements were not correctly ordered. Pastry should be served either in the main course or the sweet but not in both.

Although it was relatively easy to identify the overall structure of meals in the hospital, it was more difficult to distinguish the meaning of the meals. Douglas argued that the contrast between different meals was an important aspect of the meaning of any particular meal and the different social relations it encoded. Meals at the hospital hardly varied in structure. Even Christmas Dinner was barely different in size and structure from other meals. Where then was the contrast between different meals that gave individual meals their meaning? In one way the lack of variation in meals in the hospital when compared to meals in an ordinary household clearly differentiated institutional life from domestic life. However, the main variations were not between the pattern of meals on a ward but between the same meals on different wards. In the institution the main "message" encoded in the meals was about the nature of the relationship between the patients and their nurses.

7.3 THE CLASSIFICATION OF PATIENTS AND THE STRUCTURE OF ACTIVITIES ASSOCIATED WITH MEALS.

Nurses organised their accounts of mealtimes in terms of the grade of ward. The following extracts are taken from a written account of hospital mealtimes. Following a brief introduction, the author of the account, a nurse, described the organisation of meals on cot and chair wards.

> The meals are delivered to the wards
> ideally about half an hour before
> serving. It is preferable for the
> cot and chair wards to get theirs first
> as a fair amount of preparation has to
> be done. On the cot and chair wards the
> residents are multiply handicapped -
> very few can feed themselves
> and many cannot chew and so have only
> a semi-solid diet. When the meal arrives
> two of the staff will calculate the
> number of plates needed and then
> sub-divide them into solid diet,
> mince diet, any special diet. They will
> then serve the food onto dishes and where
> necessary cut it up. The plates are then
> loaded onto a pre-heated trolley and kept
> warm until required. While this is taking
> place, any other staff will be preparing
> the residents. Any, who are able, will
> sit up at the table and feed themselves.

Some need to be put into special chairs
and others lie on the mat with a sheet
wrapped around them for a bib. They do
not help in any way with the preparation
of the food or themselves. Most are fed
two courses and a drink and then washed.
Counting the plates ensures that nobody
gets missed out and if any are left at
the end the staff will cross check amongst
themselves to find out who.

The author of this account has described the
social relations associated with the meals in
terms of the activities associated with the nurses
and the activities associated with the patients.
The nurses played the active roles and controlled
and ordered the activities. They were the
"providers" who prepared the meals, moved the
patients to the right place and fed them. The
patients were the passive receivers. They
digested the food they were fed. It was not a
mealtime in the usual sense of the word. All the
patients did not eat the same course at the same
time. It was sequential body servicing. A
patient was fed a meal and then washed and then
the next patient was serviced.

The nurse described mealtimes on a low grade
ward in the following way:

On the "low grade" wards the majority of
patients feed themselves - thus, mealtimes
are a far speedier process. It is
possible that one of the residents will
lay the tables. All will sit up at the
tables (unless someone is particularly
disruptive). Generally one or two of the
nurses will hand out the food. Then it is
mainly supervision (ensuring that everyone
gets a chance to eat their own meals).
Those who need feeding are fed (noise
levels are kept to a minimum). Again many
of the residents are unable to communicate
verbally so the number of plates is
carefully checked. Some of them bolt
their food and either cannot or do not
chew properly and are given a mince
diet. The door through to the kitchen is
often kept locked to keep the residents
out so there is very little opportunity
for them to help with any serving etc.

> Most tend to feed themselves with spoons -
> I do not think that knives and forks are
> generally laid out.

Again the author of the account focused on
the activity pattern and social relations of the
meal. This was more like an ordinary meal. Some
of the patients were fed but most ate their meal
in the normal course structure. However, the
social relations involved were unlike those found
in a domestic meal. The nurses prepared the meal
but they did not participate in its consumption.
Instead they tried to maintain order while the
meal was being consumed. The patients ate the
meal but they did not help in preparing or
distributing the food.
The author of this account described meals on
high grade wards in the following way:

> However on high grade wards, although the
> residents do not actually serve the meals
> out they have a far greater level of
> participation in its preparation. They
> will lay the tables - help themselves to
> drinks of water - salt, sauce etc., do
> bread and butter. The majority will feed
> themselves with knives and forks and eat
> a solid diet. They will get themselves up
> to the tables - the more able helping the
> less. The meal for these people is far
> more of a social event and they are also
> able to exercise some degree of choice
> over what they actually eat and the
> amount.

Again the author described the activity
patterns associated but the emphasis was on the
extent to which these patients not only consumed
the meal but were also involved in the preparation
of the food and the social organisation of
the meal. Of the meals in the hospital, meals on
high grade wards had most in common with domestic
meals, although they were clearly differentiated
from domestic meals because there was still a
separation between the social activities of
cooking and eating. The patients did not cook the
meals and the cooks/nurses did not eat meals with
the patients.
The importance of the classification of the
patients and the meanings of this classification,

as discussed in Chapters Three to Five, were evident in this account of mealtimes in the hospital. The cot and chair patients were characterised as essentially passive with no ability to move, feed themselves, or to make their needs known. Indeed nurses were concerned that they would miss one patient and maintained checks to ensure that they did not. The low grade patients had more ability, they could move and feed themselves. However they were seen as anti-social and constantly threatened to disrupt the structure and organisation of the meal. They were seen as needing constant supervision and control. High grade patients were seen as more socially competent and more socially oriented. They were not seen as needing the rigorous social control of low grade patients. They were seen as a potential source of help in the organisation of the meal.

In the next section I shall examine how these characterisations were related to the activities at mealtimes in the hospital.

7.4 VARIATIONS IN ACTIVITY PATTERNS DURING MEALS

The account of typical meals on three different wards suggested that each involved a different pattern of activity and a different division of activities between the nurses and the patients. The account suggested that on the low grade ward, there was a rigid division of activities with staff performing all the provider activities and patients all the receiver activities. On both the cot and chair and the high grade wards this rigid division of activities broke down but in different directions. On the cot and chair wards staff performed some of the receiver activities. They had to feed the patients. On the high grade ward patients were granted special privileges to participate in the provider activities.

Preliminary observations of mealtimes indicated that they could be divided into six components. They were activities associated with:

1. Seating arrangements and sitting down;
2. The first course;
3. The second course;
4. The drinks;

5. Distribution of medication and;
6. Leaving the tables and preparing for the next activity.

Excluded from this list were laying the table and clearing the tables. These activities were excluded because they usually took place outside the main observation period and did not form an essential part of the activities on cot and chair wards. Each component activity had two possible elements:

a.   Provider activities, e.g. there was usually a sign or signal that a mealtime was about to start and that preparations should commence.

b.   Receiver activities, e.g. patients had to be placed or take their places in the "right place" so the meal could start.

In a rigid division of activities staff would perform provider activities and patients would perform receiver activities. In a flexible division, either patients would perform provider activities, e.g. a patient would indicate the mealtimes with the appropriate signal, or staff would perform activities that in normal mealtimes would be performed by someone eating the meal, e.g. moving a patient to the right place for the meal. A classification of activities usually associated with a meal is given in Table 7.1.
During my research I observed 7 meals on a low grade ward, Pelican, on a high grade ward, Seagull and on a cot and chair ward, Ravensbourn. The majority of activities on all wards followed the two sphere pattern - staff performed provider activities and patients performed receiver activities. However, on each ward there were exceptions. Table 7.2 indicates the pattern of patient involvement in provider activities and and Table 7.3 indicates the pattern of staff involvement in receiver activities. These tables only indicate the incidents in terms of meals, they do not indicate the scale on which these activities occurred. Even with this limitation a clear pattern emerged.
The low grade ward, Pelican, corresponded relatively closely to the rigid division of activities between nurses and patients. I did not record any cases of patients participating in

Mealtimes

Table   7.1   A classification   of   mealtime
activities

Provider Activities

a   Performed by staff   b   Performed by
                                  patients

1   Activities associated with seating
     arrangements

1a   Initiating meal   1bi   Initiating meal
                                1bii   Assisting other
                                         patients

2   Activities associated with the first course

2ai Serving first   2b   Handing out first
       course   course
2aii Handing out
       first course

3   Activities associated with the second course

3a   Serving second   3b   Handing out
       course   course

4   Activities associated with the drinks

4ai Serving drinks   4b   Handing out
4aii Handing out   drinks
       drinks

5   Activities associated with the distribution of
     medication

5a   Handing out drugs   5b   Helping with
                                    distribution

6   Activities associated with the end of the
     meal. Patients leaving   tables   and/or
     preparing for next activity

6a   Signalling end   6bi   Signalling end
       of the meal   of the meal
6aii Helping patients   6bii Helping patients
       to leave table   to leave table

Receiver Activities

c   Performed by patients   d   Performed by staff

1   Activities associated with seating arrangements

| 1c Patients taking places | 1d Assisting patients |

2   Activities associated with the first course

| 2c Eating first course | 2d Feeding patient first course |

3   Activities associated with the second course

| 3b Eating second course | 3d Feeding patient second course |

4   Activities associated with the drinks

| 4c Consuming drinks | 4d Feeding patients drinks |

5   Activities associated with the distribution of medication

5c Taking medication

6   Activities associated with the end of the meal. Patients leaving tables and/or preparing for next activity

| 6c Leaving tables | 6d Assisting patients to leave tables |

* This did not exhaust all possible patient performed provider activities e.g. the patients could serve the meal or feed other patients. This list was based on observations.

provider activities, despite the presence on the ward of two "high grade" patients. The nurses performed the active provider roles whereas the patients performed the passive receiver roles. I did record nurses performing receiver activities. There were three very dependent patients who had to be fed every meal.

On the high grade ward - Seagull, I recorded at least one patient performed provider activity in each meal. I recorded variations in this participation. On Day Seven participation was restricted to initiating the meal whereas on Day Four one patient even assisted in distributing drugs. A trained nurse made up the prescription and a patient handed the drugs to the relevant patient. The distribution of drugs was not only restricted to staff but also to a special category of nurses. It was one of the main duties of qualified nurses and nurses in training could only perform it, without supervision, when they had passed a special examination. On Seagull Ward there were only two examples of staff performing receiver activities.

The cot and chair ward, Ravensbourn, corresponded least to the two sphere model. Patients were not involved in and did not perform any provider activities but nurses were heavily involved in receiver activities. Only a minority of patients fed themselves. The organisation of the meal was dominated by the majority who had to be fed.

Discussion

This analysis of the division of activities provides information about the overall relationship between nurses and patients in the hospital and variations in this relationship between the three different wards. Overall, nurses dominated and controlled the patients. There was no commensality and nurses initiated the structure of meals. When patients performed provider activities, it was a privilege granted by the nurses.

The way in which this control was exercised varied on the different wards. On the low grade ward the domination took the form of a rigid division of activities. On the high grade ward nurses occasionally but not always offered (some) patients privileges. These privileged patients were allowed to perform staff activities, even help with the distribution of drugs. On the cot and chair ward nurses performed many of the receiver activities as well as all the provider activities.

The difference in the organisation of meals was undoubtedly related to the differences in abilities of patients on the three wards. However these variations in abilities did not "explain the organisation". These variations in abilities could accommodate different patterns of meals. If the organisation of meals was "determined" by patients' abilities then on high grade wards patients were capable of serving the meals - even in some cases preparing them.

The differences in the organisation of meals on the three wards was related to nurses' perceptions of patient needs as represented by grade classification of wards - "high grade" patients were seen as benefiting from a more homely environment, "low grade" patients a tough, even spartan environment and "cot and chair" patients a protective environment that provided physical care. These perceptions of needs would justify the privileges of some "high grade" patients, the rigid division of labour on "low grade" wards and the emphasis on body servicing on "cot and chair" wards. However if the organisation of meals was determined by these perceptions then one would expect a homelike environment on "high grade" wards with small groups of patients preparing and serving a meal and eating it with members of the staff.

The organisation I actually observed was a product of different strategies of control and was one way in which nurses displayed their control. This control was legitimated but not "caused" by the classifications and associated perceptions.

7.5 VARIATIONS IN THE TEMPORAL AND SPATIAL PATTERNS OF MEALS

In his study of a T.B. sanitorium, Roth showed how nurses utilised technical activities such as antisepsis as a means of maintaining practical control of the situation and the patients. They wore protective clothing only when they were working with patients, not when they were socialising, even though the risk of infection was the same:

> Apparently, these nurses believe they need
> protection only when working. They remark
> that the gown, and more especially the
> mask, is a barrier to friendly
> intercourse. (Roth: 1957, p.314)

Table 7.2 <u>Patient performed provider activities</u>*

	Pelican	Seagull	Ravensbourn
1bi		2,6,7	
1bii			
2b		2,3,4,5	
3b		1,2,3,4,5,6	
4b		4	
5b		1,5	
6bi			
6bii		4	

Table 7.3 <u>Staff performed receiver activities</u>*

	Pelican	Seagull	Ravensbourn
1d	1,2,3,4, 5,6,7	1,5	1,2,3,4,5, 6,7
2d	1,2,3,4, 5,6,7		1,2,3,4,5, 6,7
3d	1,2,3,4, 5,6,7		1,2,3,4,5, 6,7
4d	1,2,3,6, 7 **		1,2,3,4,5, 6,7
6d	1,2,3,4, 5,6,7	4,5	***

* Meals during which the activity was performed indicated by number, i.e. 2 indicates that the reported activity took place in the second observed meal.

** Drinks omitted on Pelican Ward during fourth and fifth observed meal.

*** On all the meals observed on Ravensbourn Ward the patients were left in situ after meal and had not been moved by the end of the observation period.

Rosengren and DeVault showed how hospital staff (doctors and nurses) in an obstetrical hospital utilised the physical arrangement of the unit and the timing of activities within this space to maintain their control over the patient and the situation.

> The normal circuit : admitting office, to
> prep room, to labor room, to delivery
> room, to recovery room, and finally to the
> lying-in room is adhered to scrupulously.
> The physiological tempo would often
> indicate that at least one or more rooms
> might better be forgotten, but the patient
> must adhere to this timing of movement
> from region to region, even if it means at
> a fast trot. (Rosengren and DeVault:
> 1963, p.283)

Thus an examination of the temporal and spatial activities of mealtimes should show how and in what ways meals are exploited as a means of patient control.

The Temporal Structure of Meal
Table 7.4 summarises the starting, finishing and overall times of the seven main meals on each ward. The low grade ward, Pelican, had the most rigid pattern with smallest time variations. On the high grade ward, Seagull, the meals were shorter and there was more variation in starting, finishing and overall time. Meals on Ravensbourn, the cot and chair ward, had two separate temporal patterns, one for patients who fed themselves and the other for patients who had to be fed. The meals of patients feeding themselves were similar in length to those of meals on the other wards, but there was greater variation in both starting time and finishing time. The meals of patients who had to be fed started earlier and lasted much longer than meals on the other wards.

Table 7.4 The temporal structure of meals

	Pelican	Seagull	Ravensbourn Feeders	Others
Start	11.50	11.56	12.17	11.43
Standard deviation	2.5min	3.0min	7.3min	3.9min
Finish	12.40	12.41	1.04	1.07
Standard deviation	1.9min	3.8min	5.6min	6.4min
Overall	50min	46min	47min	84min

The nurses controlled the timing of meals through their control of provider activities such as serving the meal. However occasionally nurses would display this control by making the patients sit quietly at the table. For example on Seagull Ward Meal Four started at the usual time, 11.55, but did not finish till 12.58. At 12.45 the patients had started wandering away from the tables. They were sent back by the nurse in charge who then insisted on silence. The patients sat in almost complete silence till 12.58. During this period, the nurse in charge told four patients to be quiet. The exchange with one patient went as follows:

> Nurse (to Doris) - Doris, do you want to go to O.T. this afternoon?
>
> Doris - Yes.
>
> Nurse - If you want to go you'll have to be quiet for five minutes.

The activity of this nurse during this period was expressive. She was displaying her control of the patients.

The Spatial Structure of Meals

The spatial structure of meals was evident in the seating arrangements. On the ambulant wards, the majority of patients sat at tables (a maximum of four to each table). These tables were in a dining area at the end of the dayroom. The places were allocated by nurses and only occasionally changed. On the cot and chair wards patients ate and were fed in a variety of places. The more able patients ate their meals sitting at a table. The rest were fed in geriatric chairs, wheelchairs, on bean bags, sitting on the floor or lying on the mat. There were no fixed places, even for the more able patients.

On Ravensbourn Ward patients at the two extremes of competence, the elderly patients or "geriatrics" who could feed themselves sat at a table and most of the difficult "non-feeders" were fed on a mat. Both the table and the mat were in the middle of the room. The other non-feeders were fed in wheelchairs or chairs arranged along the walls of the dayroom. (See Diagram 7.1)

Mealtimes

Diagram **7.1** <u>Spatial location of patient groups during mealtimes on Ravensbourn Ward</u>.

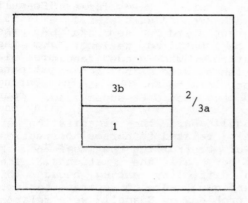

<u>Code</u>

1. "Geriatrics"
2/3a. Intermediate and very dependent patients
3b. The difficult feeders or "mat patients"

On the two ambulant wards space was organised in a different way. Most tables were in a dining area at the end of the dayroom. On Seagull Ward two tables were placed at the other end of the dayroom and formed a separate dining area for the elderly patients. On Pelican two "non feeders" were fed in geriatric chairs. The trays attached to these tables prevented the non feeders wandering and disrupting other patients. On both wards patients sat at the same table for each meal. On Seagull patients sat in the same seats, on Pelican they sat at the same table but staff occasionally put patients in the "wrong" chairs. Although the use of space on the cot and chair wards and the ambulant wards was different, both types of spatial organisation were related to the overall organisation of the meal. On the cot and chair ward most patients were fed in sequence. Therefore arranging the majority along the "edges" of the dayroom allowed staff to move round and feed patients in order. Two groups needed different treatment. The "feeders" sat at tables and fed themselves. Nurses could provide them with food and then leave them to eat it. The difficult feeders were also separated as they took much longer to feed. Separating the difficult feeders from the others allowed for a "fairer" distribution of work amongst ward staff.

On the low grade ward two separate "problem" subgroups could be identified, patients who were difficult and patients who needed feeding. On Pelican these patients were either separated from other patients or located in the middle of the dining area where they could be supervised. (See Diagram 7.2).

On the Seagull Ward the organisation of mealtimes was again related to nurses' perception of difficulties of controlling the meal and of providing food for all the patients. The patients who had difficulty eating, because of their physical handicaps, were on separate tables. The behavioural problems on Seagull were related to intergroup relations, especially the relationships between the older group of patients and the younger active patients. These two groups were separated. The older group were given their own separate dining area at the end of the dayroom. (See Diagram 7.3). There was one anomaly, the patients who caused much of the friction between the two groups were seated at the same table.

Discussion

This section has examined the temporal and spatial organisation of mealtimes on three wards. The staff determined both the temporal and spatial organisation of the meal, and the organisation therefore reflected staff perception of problems. On the low grade ward the emphasis was on patient control. There was a rigid well defined time pattern with little daily variation. The problem patients were centrally located where they could be more easily serviced and controlled. On the high grade ward the same time and spatial framework existed but with more variation. The control of patients was socially oriented rather than individualistic.

The organisation of both time and space on the two ambulant wards was different from that on the cot and chair ward. On the ambulant ward the social dimension of mealtimes, however reduced, was still evident. On the cot and chair ward, it

Diagram 7.2 The spatial location of patient groups during mealtime on Pelican Ward

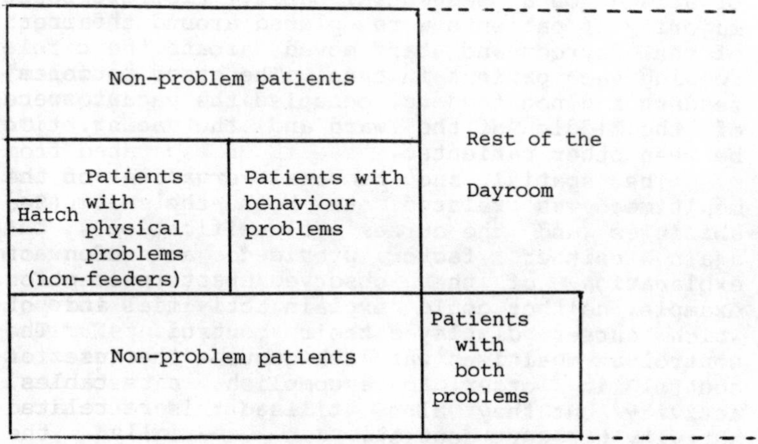

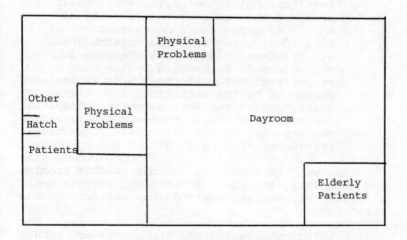

Diagram 7.3 The spatial location of patient groups during mealtimes on Seagull Ward

would be more accurate to describe mealtimes as feeding times. The emphasis was on routine body servicing of patients. This body servicing was organised on a sequential basis. Therefore the majority of patients were placed around the edges of the dayroom and staff moved around the circle feeding each patient in turn. The other patients, feeders and non feeders, occupied the vacant space of the middle of the ward and the vacant time between other patients.

The spatial and temporal organisation of mealtimes was related to both the patients' abilities and the nurses' classifications, but again neither factor provided an adequate explanation of the observed patterns. For example, neither could explain activities through which nurses displayed their control. Nurses' control at mealtimes was ambiguous - they exerted control in order to accomplish a technical activity but they also utilised this technical activity to exert control.

The first part of this analysis has been generally accepted. For example, Freidson wrote:

> For the job (of treating illness in institutions) to be performed at all requires some administrative routine, and it requires the reduction of individual patients to administrative and treatment classes, all members in each class to be managed by the same set of routines. If the job is to be performed to the satisfaction of the staff, procedures that minimise inter-ferences with their routine and maximise their convenience are required. (Freidson: 1975, p.312)

However the ambiguous nature of this control and especially the use of technical activities as a method of social control has attracted less attention.

7.5   VARIATIONS IN INTERACTION PATTERNS DURING MEALS: QUALITATIVE DATA

In the introduction to this chapter, I argued that meals not only have an overt biological function, providing nourishment for the patients, but they also provide information about

interpersonal relations. In the third section of
this chapter I examined the division of activities
at mealtimes and showed that nurses dominated.
Nurses served the meal, patients ate it. In the
fourth section I examined the temporal and spatial
organisation of meals. On all three wards staff
used both time and space to maintain control over
the meal and over the patients. Each meal not
only consisted of a set of technical activities
accomplished within a spatial and temporal
framework but also of a set of verbal (and
physical) interactions. There were important
qualitative and quantitative variations in the
interaction patterns between the three wards. In
this section I shall examine qualitative data on
the variations in the interaction patterns and in
the next section quantitative data.

On all three wards the main volume of verbal
interaction was concerned with the technical
activities of the meal, and maintaining staff
control. On both Pelican and Seagull Wards the
interaction was between staff and patients,
whereas on Ravensbourn the interaction was between
the nurses. Staff/patient interactions on
Ravensbourn were limited to the physical acts of
feeding.

On the low grade ward the staff/patient
interactions took the form of a series of
instructions and commands. The majority of these
were directed at the patients who were disrupting
or threatening to disrupt the meal. The following
record is a good example of the difficult
behaviour of Vicky, the attempts of ward staff to
control it and the consequence of verbal
interaction between Vicky and the nurses, for
other patients on her table, Jean, Angela and
Moira.

> (At 12.06 the majority of the patients were
> sitting at the table. Vicky is still
> dancing by the radio. Nurse S, who is
> new to the ward, tries to get her to sit
> down.)
>
> Nurse S - What's your name?
>
> Vicky - (No reply).
>
> Nurse S - Come on, won't you show me your
> place? (Vicky carries on dancing so

Nurse S turns to Nurse A.)

Nurse S - I can't get that patient to sit
    down. (Nurse A takes no notice and
    Vicky carries on dancing. At 12.10
    Nurse A turns her attention to Vicky.)

Nurse A - Vicky! Vicky! Come on.
    (Vicky doesn't move so Nurse A walks
    across the dayroom and takes her hand.)

Vicky - No! No!
    (Nurse A switches off the radio. Vicky
    runs over and switches it on. Nurse A
    switches it off and removes the plug.)

Nurse A - Vicky, sit down.
    (All the other patients at Vicky's
    table look apprehensive. Moira holds
    up her hands as if to defend herself.
    Jean shifts her chair away from the table.
    Angela stands up.)

Nurse A - Vicky! Sit down!
    (Vicky sits down and pinches Moira twice.)

Nurse A - Stop it, Vicky.
    (Vicky pinches Moira again. Gets up and
    walks towards Katie a severely handicapped
    defenceless patient. She is pushed back
    to her chair by Nurse A. Vicky again
    pinches Moira. Jean moves her chair right
    away. Vicky gets up and pulls Nurse A's
    hair. Nurse A pushes her back in her
    seat. Ruth starts crying, is upset.
    Nurse A comes to clear the plates from the
    table. Vicky pinches her. Jean runs
    down to the toilets. Vicky scratches
    Angela. None of the nurses notice.
    Angela starts smacking her own head.)

Nurse S - Angela stop it.
    (Ruth Barker walks over and hits Vicky
    on the head with a spoon.)

Nurse A - Ruth, leave her alone.
    (Nurse A stands over the table to
    supervise for a minute. When her back
    is turned Vicky gets up and attacks
    Kay, a wheelchair patient.)

Nurse D - Vicky, what are you doing?
(Vicky goes back to her table and starts
eating her pudding - tinned pears.
She also takes some from Moira's plate.
She eats her pears with her hand.
Having finished her own pears, she turns
her attention to Angela's but Nurse A
notices.)

Nurse A - Vicky, it wasn't yours, was it?
(Nurse A puts the tinned pears back
on Angela's plate then clears all the
plates off the table except Angela's.
Moira is also trying to steal Angela's.
pears. Vicky gets up and comes over to me.
She tries to poke my eyes but I avoid her.
She then sits down. The meal ends.
Vicky goes to the toilets with the rest.
She then comes into the dayroom. The
radio has been plugged in. She switches
it on and starts dancing.)

(Pelican Meal Five)

The interaction was about control. It was
initiated because Vicky had failed to respond to
an earlier generalised instruction to all the
patients and therefore needed an individual
specific instruction. Both nurses attempted to
control Vicky verbally at first and then resorted
to physical control. Vicky redirected her
behaviour into physical aggression against
patients on her table and other vulnerable
patients. A chain reaction developed. The
incident was terminated by the end of the meal,
when Vicky returned to her favourite pastime.
On Seagull Ward the majority of staff/patient
interaction was again concerned with the control
of the meal, but the methods of control were more
socially oriented. Sarcasm and public ridicule
were used rather than physical force. The
following extract also shows how the more able
patients (in this case Linda) were used to care
for the most dependent patients.

(All the patients are seated waiting
for the meal to be handed out. The
nurse in charge, Nurse R, checks that
all patients are ready and notices that
the messy feeders don't have any sheets

on. Bed sheets are used as bibs.)

Nurse R - Where are the sheets then?

Greta - There aren't any.

Nurse R - There must be some. Matron,
(Linda's nickname) go and have a look
in the linen cupboard.
(Linda goes out of the dayroom and comes
back with four sheets. She drapes them
round four patients, Pat, Susan, Jean
and Moira. The first course is handed
out. Pat finds it difficult to eat
and pulls her sheet up.)

Nurse R - Who put Girlie's (Pat's nickname)
sheet on?

Greta and others - Linda.

Nurse R - Matron, can't you do any better
than that? Look it is all round her
shoulders and there's nothing round
her front. She's dropping all her food
down her front. Matron, put it right.
(Linda gets up and adjusts the sheet.)

(Seagull Meal Five)

On Seagull Ward there were also more
symmetrical interactions between staff and
patients, often initiated by the patients. In the
following extract Greta initiated a conversation
with me and with the nurse in charge.

Greta - It's a nice meal, Andy.

Andy - What is it?

Greta - I think it is pork. Jenny (nurse in
charge) what is it?

Nurse J - Pork.

Greta - (Laughs) You can write that down in
your book.

(Seagull Meal Six)

On the cot and chair ward the interaction was about rather than with the patients. Patients were treated as passive recipients and the exchanges between staff were about how, or in what order, patients should be fed and interaction between staff increased as the meal progressed. As the number of patients left to be fed decreased so did the number and variety of remaining meals, therefore the need to check and match unfed patients with remaining diets increased. The following extract is an example of the interchanges that took place towards the end of one meal on Ravensbourn.

> (Nurse R finishes feeding Peter and looks
> for next patient to be fed.)
> Nurse R - Has Snow been done?
>
> Nurse J - No.
> (Nurse R goes to the heated meal trolley
> and looks for a meal for Robert Snow.)
>
> Nurse R - You've done it again Jean.
> (Nurse J served out the meals.)
> There aren't enough dinners.
>
> Physiotherapist G - There's Robert and
> two others still to be fed.
>
> Nurse R - There are only two dinners.
> (Nurse R fetches an extra plate from
> the kitchen and divides the two remaining
> dinners into three.)
>
> Nurse J - There's a lot of pudding left in
> the liquidiser.
>
> (Ravensbourn Meal One)

With the ordinary feeders who sat along the wall of the dayroom , nurses were interested in the sequence of feeding and matching patients to diet. These problems increased and therefore staff/staff interaction rose as staff neared the end of the circle. The remaining patients' occupying the central space of the dayroom, presented a different problem. Nurses had to decide how and when they should be fitted into the main sequence. This problem had to be resolved at each meal, hence the variation in the mealtimes of the "feeders". This negotiation is clear in the following interstaff interaction.

> (Nurse L prepared the meal for the old ones who are sitting at the tables waiting. The rest of the nurses are sitting on the mat feeding the difficult ones.)
>
> Nurse R (to Nurse L) - Do one of the difficult ones.
>
> Nurse L - If Cathy (a nurse) does Susie then all the difficult ones will be done.
>
> Nurse R - Do Belinda.
>
> Nurse L - O.K. That is the second time today I'll have done Belinda.
> (Nurse L leaves the old ones' meals and feeds Belinda. Half an hour later he returns to the meals trolley. He comments to me.)
>
> Nurse L - They've (the old ones) fallen asleep waiting for me.
>
> (Ravensbourn Meal Five.)

Discussion

The interaction pattern on the three wards was related to the nurses' control of the meal. On the three wards the content of the interaction varied according to the dominant problem of the meal. On the low grade ward, the physical control of patients was seen as the greatest problem and the content of interaction with patients was predominantly instructions and orders. On the high grade ward, there were fewer problems of control. Indeed nurses used the patients to assist them in the meal. Although interaction was also in the form of instructions and orders, the tone was less peremptory and the orientation was social rather than individual. Nurses responded to the social interactions initiated by patients. On the cot and chair ward there was little staff/staff patient interaction. Nurses treated patients as passive objects to be serviced. The main interactions between the staff were about the order and sequence of the body servicing - when to do the patients outside the main circle and how the main circle was progressing.

7.6   VARIATIONS   IN   INTERACTION   PATTERNS   DURING MEALS: QUANTITATIVE DATA

In   my   records   of   meals,   I   concentrated on   the   main   activities   and   associated interactions.   I   treated other   interactions   as background   noise,   noting   the general   direction, e.g.   who   was   gossiping   to   whom   but   not   the detailed   content.   My   records   were   therefore limited. Given   these limitations,   in   my   analysis of this   data I   shall   exclude   all non-functional interactions and   concentrate   on   the quantitative analysis of functional interactions.

I   did not   use   precoded   categories   for   my observations   but   recorded   who   was   involved   in interactions   and   as   much   as   possible   of   the content   of   the   interactions.   Therefore   in the analysis   of   the   data on   interactions during meals I   needed   to   classify these   records. Since nurses   dominated the   structure   of   the meal,   I focused   on   their   pattern   of   interactions   and classified them   into three categories.

* Unequal nurse/patient interactions, e.g. a nurse ordering patients;

* Equal nurse/patient interactions, e.g. patients asking a nurse a question and the nurse responding;

* Nurse/nurse interactions about the patients;   e.g. nurses talking about the patients.

The   volume   of   verbal   interactions   during mealtimes   was   generally   low,   furthermore interactions between nurses and patients tended to attract the attention of all the patients so there was   often only   one   major   exchange   to   observe. There was   usually   no   problem   in   classifying interactions as nurses clearly signalled different types of   interaction with   the tone of their voice and   the   loudness   with which   they   spoke.   For example orders were usually issued in a loud, firm voice.

These three interaction   patterns can be seen as the interactional equivalent of the three types of activity patterns. The dominance   pattern was the   interactional equivalent of the rigid division of   activities.   The   equality   pattern   was   the interactional equivalent of patients performing provider activities and the interstaff pattern was the interactional equivalent of the activity pattern in which staff perform receiver activities such as feeding the patients.

The interaction patterns of the three wards are shown on Table 7.5. The interactions follow the predicted, and by now, familiar pattern. On Pelican and Seagull Wards, the volume of interactions was similar but the pattern different. The rigid two sphere activity pattern, on Pelican, was associated with nurses giving orders to patients, an unequal dominance pattern of interaction. On Seagull Ward, the increased participation of patients in the meal was associated with a more equal pattern of interaction. On Ravensbourn Ward, the increased involvement of nurses in the receiver activities was associated with an interstaff pattern of communication. The patients were the passive objects of the communications rather than the active subjects. The individualistic body servicing on Ravensbourn was associated with a lower overall level of communication. Although meals on Ravensbourn were nearly twice as long, there were only half the recorded number of interactions.

Table 7.5 <u>Interaction patterns on the three wards during seven mealtimes</u> (Percentage figures are percentages of all interactions on the ward)

	Pelican	Seagull	Ravensbourn
Unequal	58 (66%)	37 (43%)	12 (25%)
Equal	20 (23%)	42 (48%)	11 (23%)
Staff/Staff	10 (11%)	8 (9%)	25 (52%)
Total	88	87	48

Coser, in her study on hospital care, also recorded interaction patterns (Coser: 1963). Although she did not use the same categories nor concentrate on the interaction patterns associated with any specific activity, there were certain points of similarity between the two studies. Coser classified interactions into three categories:

1. Staff acting on patients without
    eliciting response, i.e. nonverbal
    interaction;

2. Verbal staff/patient interactions;

3. Verbal staff/staff interaction.

Coser treated all verbal staff/patient interactions as equivalent whereas I analysed my records of staff/patient interactions in two distinctive classes. Furthermore I excluded nonfunctional staff/staff interactions. However in my records I also included nonverbal interaction, i.e. staff acting on patients. Therefore there was a point of direct comparison between Coser's study and my own.

In both studies there are similar patterns of interactions. Wards with a high percentage of staff/staff interactions were also the wards on which staff acted on patients without eliciting response. These were wards in which staff concentrated on body servicing of the patients (See Table 7.6).

Coser concentrated on the staff/staff interaction pattern and built her hypothesis on the basis of these patterns. She argued that there was a relationship between interaction patterns and resource allocation. Coser hypothesised that the lower the resources (in terms of available staff) or the more difficult the task (in terms of patient dependency), the more nurses and other professionals would withdraw from the main care task and the patients. Therefore, as resources fell or work increased, there would be a fall in the overall rate of interaction accompanied by a rise in the percentage of interactions taking place between staff.

> An acute shortage of personnel does not
> necessarily increase each person's
> load; it may get so bad that it
> legitimizes withdrawal from the task.
> (Coser: 1963, p.247)

This observation led her to postulate that:

181

Table 7.6 <u>Relationship between staff acting on patient and staff to staff interactions.</u>

<u>Jane Eagle Study</u>

Ward	Staff acting on patients	Staff to staff interaction
Seagull	16	8
Pelican	199	10
Ravensbourn	322	25
Total	537	43

<u>Coser's Study</u>

Center	9	25
Active Treatment	27	29
Long-term Treatment	21	27
Custodial	48	66
Total	105	147

> the greater the number of patients in relation to nurses in a ward, the more staff tend to spend time among themselves. (Coser: 1963, p.246)

Although Coser's evidence supported her hypothesis, the material from the Jane Eagle Hospital does not (see Diagram 7.4). In Coser's study as staff resources fell and the patient nurse ratio rose so the level of staff/staff interaction rose. Observation of meal oriented interactions at the Jane Eagle Hospital showed a reverse relationship. Staff/staff interaction rose as staff resources rose.

There were, of course, important differences between the studies in terms of patients (physically ill v mentally handicapped), staffing levels (Coser's wards exhibited a far greater variation in staffing levels) and type of observations (Coser used all interactions whereas

Mealtimes

Diagram 7.4 A comparison of the relationship between interaction patterns and staffing ratios between Jane Eagle and R. Coser's observations.
(Coser: 1963, Table II)

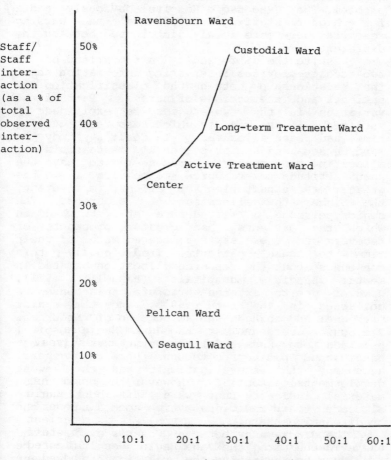

Staff/
Staff
inter-
action
(as a % of
total
observed
inter-
action)

50%   Ravensbourn Ward
                    Custodial Ward

40%   Long-term Treatment Ward
              Active Treatment Ward
          Center
30%

20%
      Pelican Ward
          Seagull Ward
10%

0   10:1   20:1   30:1   40:1   50:1   60:1

Patient-Nurse Ratio
(Number of patients per nurse per shift)
Falling Resources ─────────────>

I concentrated on functional interactions). However Coser's hypothesis was obviously intended to apply to different institutions and I am comparing the trends of interactions rather than interactions per se. However the variations in overall staffing levels presented a greater problem. The Jane Eagle Hospital obviously had a far higher staffing level and the nursing resources were more evenly distributed between the different wards.

Despite the differences, a comparison of the two studies provides interesting information about the relationship between the classification of patients and the actions of nurses. Part of the variation in the two studies is explained by variations in the way in which resources (nursing time) had been allocated. In Coser's study the ward nurses and senior personnel responsible for allocating resources to wards seemed to have the same attitude to resource allocation, i.e. the greater the expectation of patient improvement, the higher the allocation of resources. The senior personnel allocated more staff to wards in which the patients had greater prospects of recovery and these staff allocated more of their time to these patients. Traditionally this consensus about the resource allocation existed in mental handicap hospitals (Hassell: 1971). However, due to external pressure, this consensus collapsed in the late 60's, and the senior personnel had changed the allocation of resources. The senior personnel at the Jane Eagle Hospital provided more nurses for the wards with the most handicapped patients although there was general agreement that these patients had the lowest developmental potential. However the observation material indicated that ward staff continued to allocate their individual time according to the traditional pattern.

The discrepancy between Coser's evidence and the evidence from the Jane Eagle Hospital can be resolved by examining the relationship between nurses' descriptions of the patients' developmental potential and interaction patterns rather than the relationship between staffing levels and interaction patterns. Coser suggested there was a major difference between nurses' attitudes to patients at the Center and on the Sunnydale Wards. The Center nurses expected improvement and discharge. "All Center nurses mention the goal of restoring patients to the community" (Coser: 1963, p.234). The Sunnydale nurses did not expect their patients to leave. The names Coser gave to the Sunnydale wards suggested a gradation from nonimprovement on the Active Treatment and Long Term Treatment wards to deterioration on the Custodial Ward. Some of the terms nurses used to describe patients on the Custodial Ward, were similar to those used by nurses in the Jane Eagle Hospital to describe "cot and chair" patients, e.g. "this is considered the end of the road, and people here talk of them as vegetables" (Coser: 1963, p.234). Thus in Coser's study and the Jane Eagle study, we can divide nurses' description of the patients' developmental potential into three categories:

* patients' condition likely to improve, the Center and Seagull Ward;

* patients' condition likely to remain the same, Active and Long Term Treatment Wards and Pelican Ward;

* patients' condition likely to deteriorate, Custodial Ward and Ravensbourn Ward.

These perceptions appeared to be related to nurses' allocation of their own time to different groups of patients.

Discussion

A reexamination of Table 7.6 suggests a different explanation to the one offered by Coser. On Seagull Ward (and the Center) staff were willing to talk to the patients, and spent less time interacting with each other or acting on the patients. On Pelican (and the Active and Long Term Treatment Wards) higher dependency levels were associated with a rise in staff acting on patients. On Ravensbourn Ward (and Custodial Ward) the individualised body servicing of patients was associated with both higher levels of staff acting on patients and staff to staff interactions. Thus rather than withdrawal from the task the interaction patterns observed at the Jane Eagle were associated with the different strategies of patient care adopted on different wards.

7.7 CONCLUSION

This chapter has examined the organisation (division of labour, temporal and spatial structure and interaction patterns) of one activity in the hospital, eating.

If the hospital meal is treated as a message, then, within the organisation of meals, there were a variety of messages. At the overall level, the common features of meals indicated that nurses controlled and dominated patients. There was no commensality and the staff determined what was eaten and how it was eaten. Nurses controlled the division of labour and the temporal and spatial structure of mealtimes. This structure and its pattern of relations clearly signalled that these were institutional not domestic meals.

Within this overall message, there were specific messages related to different wards. Nurses used different strategies of control on the different wards.

On the high grade ward, Seagull, meals were more relaxed. There was evidence that nurses were more indulgent to the patients and allowed them (within limits) to adjust the content and style of the meal to suit their individual tastes and social relations. Patients were treated as more competent and equal. They were allowed to perform some of the provider activities, even activities such as drug distribution associated with high status among the nurses. The temporal structure of the meals was more varied. Space was used as a control mechanism but one aspect of control involved the social relations amongst the patients. Although the analysis of interactions was limited to functional interactions, the quality and quantity of these interactions indicated a more equal relationship between nurses and patients. Orders were phrased as requests and the conventions of interactions between equals were generally maintained. This organisation was consistent with nurses' typification of high grade patients as socially oriented persons who required a more personalised environment.

On the low grade ward, Pelican, the patients were treated as physical individuals not social groups. There was a rigid division of labour. The nurses performed the provider roles and the patients, except for a small minority, performed the receiver roles. The time structure was rigid with little variation. Space was used for the control of individuals not groups. The interactions during meals were directly concerned with patient control and were dominated by unequal nurse/patient interactions. This structure was consistent with nurse typifications of low grade patients as physically active anti-social individuals who need physical control.

On the cot and chair ward, Ravensbourn, the patients were treated as "mere organisms" that required body servicing. Nurses performed most of the activities, both the provider and the receiver activities. The individualised body servicing meant that all the patients, except the "feeders" were individually fed. Each patient was fed the whole meal before the nurse moved on to the next patient. The temporal, spatial and interaction patterns were all determined by the routine body servicing of the patients. The more competent patients who could feed themselves and the difficult feeders were fitted into the space and time left by the other patients. The meals on Ravensbourn were also the most varied in time and space structure. The nurses adjusted the structure of each meal to fit the particular social relations between nurses on duty. This fitted with the nurse typification of patients as physical objects who required servicing but who had few if any social needs.

There was, therefore, a clear relationship between nurses' characterisations of the patients, patients' abilities and the way in which nurses organised meals on different wards. However it was neither a simple nor a causal relationship. Patients' abilities did not result in a certain type of organisation nor did they explain the different organisation of meals on the different wards. There was a degree of overlap in terms of ability between the different wards. For example, there were several patients on Pelican Ward who were more like cot and chair patients than other low grade patients and there was a group of elderly patients on Ravensbourn Ward who were more like low grade than cot and chair patients. The "cot and chair" patients on Pelican did not receive sequential body servicing and the treatment of elderly patients on the cot and chair ward was very different to the treatment of patients on the two ambulant wards. The abilities of the patients on different wards undoubtedly set limits to the organisation of meals. The heavily dependent cot and chair patients had to be fed, but these abilities did not determine which particular pattern was selected, e.g. cot and chair patients could be fed in the dormitory on their beds or cots or in the dayroom on mats etc., or each patient could be fed a complete meal or all the patients could be fed one course first.

I have argued that the organisation of meals was related to the nurses' classification of wards and the perceptions associated with these classifications, e.g. that high grade patients need a homely environment. However the classification did not provide a complete explanation. More especially it could not be used to explain the ambiguous nature of control at mealtimes - meals were used as a way of establishing and maintaining control but control was also a means to an end, getting the patients fed. I would suggest that the classification of patients did not result in a certain organisation of meals but legitimated the organisation adopted by nurses. Freidson's analysis of the relationship between control or power and staff attitudes in an activity/passivity relationship (a relationship in which staff act without considering the wishes of the patient) would fit the situation described in this chapter.

> The exercise of power to overcome resistance when the patient is not in a coma is legitimized by the social identity imputed to the patient : he is just an infant, a cat, a retardate, a psychotic, or in some other way not fully human and responsible and so cannot be allowed to exercise his own choice to withdraw from treatment. (Freidson: 1975, p.318)

The actual organisation was determined by the staff need or desire to control the patient and was legitimated by the social identity imputed in the classification.

CHAPTER 8
NURSES' CONTROL STRATEGIES: THREE CASE STUDIES

8.1 INTRODUCTION

In Chapter Seven I examined the organisation
of meals on three wards. I showed that although
the different routines adopted by nurses on the
three wards were consistent with nurses'
expectations of patients on each ward, these
expectations did not "cause" the routines rather
they legitimated them. They legitimated the
nurses' control of the organisation of the meals
and of patient behaviour during meal times.

As meals were important activities in the
hospital, they set the rhythm of the organisation.
Each day was very much like every other in terms
of meals and on each ward one meal was like the
next. Meal times created a cyclical time that
structured the activities of, and interactions
between, groups of patients and groups of staff.
Bloch has developed the concept of cyclical time
to describe the pattern underlying ritual
activity. He suggested that each culture has its
own special cyclical time which forms the basis of
ritual activities. His suggestion that ritual
serves to conceal domination has obvious parallels
with my analysis as I have suggested that the
routine of basic care activities conceals
domination. He contrasted cyclical time with
durational time that is used for practical
activities such as agriculture. He argued that
durational time is common to different cultures
(Bloch: 1977, and Bourdillon: 1978).

It would, however, be a mistake to suggest
that nurses and other members of staff were not
aware of the individuality of the patients.
Although patients might be denied full adult

189

Control Strategies

status and therefore an independent social
identity, this did not mean that nurses were
unaware of the uniqueness of each patient (Mauss:
1979b, pp.57-94). Patients could and did stand
apart from the group. They could do this in a
variety of ways but the most common was refusal to
follow the ward routine. This refusal was a
challenge to the authority of the nurses and
required from the nurses both explanations and
action - explanations, because their ideology that
the meals were provided for the benefit of the
patients was challenged and action, because their
practical control was challenged.
    The type of threat posed varied between the
three classes of ward. On the cot and chair wards
most of the patients were so handicapped that few
had the ability or resources to upset the routine.
On low grade wards patients had the physical
ability to disrupt but their lack of social
skills, especially their inability to talk and
explain why they were being difficult, meant that
they did not challenge the ideological basis of
nurses' authority and the use of routine methods
of control needed little or no justification. On
the high grade wards patients had the ability not
only to be uncooperative, they could also talk
about their situation. They could therefore
challenge the ideological basis of authority in
the hospital. They could express a desire for
autonomy and independence that was difficult to
deny yet had to be denied because life in an
institution was regimented.
    In this chapter I shall examine these control
strategies through a case study approach (Strauss
and Glaser: 1970). I shall examine the care and
control of three high grade patients. I have
ordered my cases in terms of ability and social
competence. My first case, Denise, was the least
able of the three. Although she could talk her
comprehension and memory seemed limited. Therefore
nurses were able to discount her statements.
However Denise was, at the time of my research, a
comparatively new admission, therefore her
problems generated a lot of discussion. I have
recorded some of this discussion and I examine the
relationship between it and the ways in which
nurses dealt with Denise. My second case, Alison,
was more able than Denise. She could talk about
her situation in a coherent fashion. It was more
difficult to discount her statements. Alison had

190

had a long institutional history, therefore her problems did not generate the same level of discussion as Denise's. The explanations of Alison's behaviour were well established and well documented. However it was still possible to examine the relationship between these explanations and the patterns of control adopted by staff. Eva was the most able of the three. She was a widow and she had a son. Although she was probably easier to control than either Denise or Alison, the intellectual problems she posed were more complex.

8.2 DENISE

Introduction

During my research at the Jane Eagle Hospital, Denise lived on Seagull Ward. She was about 30 years old and had had a relatively complex career. She had lived at home until her mother died when she was 27. For the next three years she was variously cared for by her relatives, at a local authority hostel, and in a small mental handicap unit attached to a district general hospital. None of these arrangements had proved satisfactory and Denise was finally admitted, as a last resort, to Seagull Ward.

The staff at the hospital found Denise a difficult and demanding patient and in this case study I examine the ways in which they treated Denise. I have divided the case study into three parts; in the first I discuss the main problems associated with Denise's care; in the second explanations offered by different participants; and in the third the strategies adopted to control Denise and to minimise the problems she created for the hospital staff.

Problems at the Jane Eagle Hospital

The problems associated with Denise's care fell into three main areas; the problems created by her diabetes and the associated problems of her daily care; the problems associated with Denise's talk; and the problems associated with Denise's relatives.

Problems of Daily Care

Denise suffered from diabetes. She frequently had very low blood-sugar levels and there was a constant danger of hypoglycaemic attacks. Her refusal to follow

the routine created problems in the management of
her diabetes. The ward charge nurse described the
situation in the following way:

> She's one of the problem patients. Clinical
> problem diabetes. She'll often flatly
> refuse meals. She often hoards food at
> mealtimes. Sometimes makes herself vomit
> after a meal. She buys food with sugar in
> at the canteen ... She hides herself in
> the hospital, especially in the ward at
> meal times.

Denise refused to follow the normal ward
routine. For example on weekdays, the majority of
Seagull patients attended the occupational therapy
unit. Denise would often leave the ward with the
other patients but sometimes would not go to the
unit or would return to the ward. She was also
reluctant to eat her meals with the other
patients. If she did not eat her meals or take
her medication then her physical condition could
rapidly deteriorate.

Denise not only rejected the organisational
rules but also avoided relationships with other
patients. This refusal to associate with other
patients was related to her failure to follow the
routine. As Denise avoided the majority of other
patients, she often missed the cues that indicated
the start of routine activities.

Problems associated with Denise's stories Denise's
use of language appeared to be good. She had an
extensive vocabulary and her sentence construction
was good. She used this ability to accuse the
nurses of maltreatment. One such accusation was
recorded in the ward notes in the following way:

> Denise arrived at the Administration Block
> making vague complaints about nursing
> staff on the ward: These complaints
> involved night staff giving her a cup of
> tea and waking her up too early. Also
> included in complaints was a statement
> that Staff Nurse R. had hit her over the
> head.

These accusations could and did create
mistrust amongst the different groups responsible
for Denise's care. The accusation recorded above

resulted in an investigation by senior hospital
staff which was inconclusive. A similar
situation occurred when Denise was admitted to
the local general hospital for investigation of
her diabetes. The ward charge nurse described the
incident in the following way:

> When she went to the General Hospital she
> told them some fantastic stories about
> us ... that we wouldn't give her break-
> fast, we took her glasses away and that
> she was crawling round the floor on her
> hands and knees looking for her breakfast.
> It's in her medical notes. When they got
> her at the General Hospital they found her
> extremely lovable. When she came back
> the story she came out with was that they
> tied her to the bed, the nurses beat her
> up, and the matron, the one with the big
> hat, came round and jumped on her.

A major area of tension created by Denise's
stories was between the ward staff and Denise's
relatives. Ward staff were antagonised by
Denise's statements that her relatives encouraged
her to break hospital rules.

Problems with Denise's relatives The relationship
between Denise's relatives and hospital staff
could be described as one of mutual distrust. A
major source of conflict was the arrangements for
home leave. Prior to Denise's admission, her
relatives requested hospital transport for home
leave. The Jane Eagle Hospital was about 20 miles
from their home. The consultant recorded the
relatives' request for transport and her reasons
for refusing it.

> Mr. D. accepted hospital care for Denise on
> a trial basis, at the same time expressing
> his disappointment and also his intention
> that none of the family will continue to
> take Denise home for weekend leave unless
> transport is provided. As each of the
> three members of the family to whom Denise
> goes owns a car, I pointed out to Mr. D.
> that I felt this was unreasonable.

For three months following Denise's
admission, the relatives collected Denise. Then

the following incident was recorded:

> An ambulance arrived to take Denise home
> today at about 4.30 p.m. Pharmacy -
> closed. No request received for weekend
> leave. Denise herself did not know.
> Apparently this is a weekly booking to
> take her home. Ambulance driver phoned
> the headquarters and was told that the
> booking was made by Dr. N. (G.P.).

Following this incident Denise was collected
regularly by the ambulance service.

Following Denise's original admission to care
there had been constant conflict between the staff
and her relatives over her treatment. This reached
its highest pitch during Denise's stay at the
general hospital mental handicap unit. The
consultant finally lost his patience when the
relatives questioned his treatment of her
diabetes.

> Denise's relatives telephone me at home and
> the sister was extremely rude on the phone
> demanding that I changed the insulin
> dosage and pointing out that as far as she
> was concerned she knew more about diabetes
> and Denise's condition than anybody else,
> and, therefore, she should regulate the
> dosage. I informed her that if she was
> not satisfied with the treatment she
> should take Denise home and look after her
> herself and there was no reason why she
> could not collect her at any time ...

At the Jane Eagle there were no formal
complaints by the relatives but there was obvious
tension between the hospital staff and Denise's
relatives.

<u>Summary of Problems</u>   Denise presented hospital
staff with a multitude of problems.   She refused
to follow the ward routine thereby disrupting the
smooth running of the ward and threatening her own
well being.   She accused different individuals of
maltreatment and this created mistrust between the
various groups responsible for her care.   Her
relatives constantly challenged the competence of
hospital personnel.   From the point of view of
the nurses on Seagull Ward, these problems

could be grouped into two categories: the practical problems, e.g. getting Denise to eat a proper diet and getting Denise in the right place at the right time; and the intellectual problems. Both Denise and her relatives challenged the competence and integrity of the hospital staff.

At the time of my research Denise was a recent admission to the Jane Eagle Hospital and her problems attracted a lot of interest and discussion. During these discussions different participants offered different explanations and suggested different solutions. I shall examine these in the next section.

Different Interpretations of the Situation

Participants' interpretations of Denise's problems were based on their theories of the causes of this behaviour. There were several competing and sometimes conflicting theories that broadly fell into 6 categories: the relatives'; the traditional medical; the progressive medical; the psychologist's; the social worker's and the nurses'. The theories aimed to explain the problems. They differed in the relative emphasis they gave to different aspects of the situation.

The Relatives' View   I could not be certain about the relatives' view as one of the conditions of my study was that I should not contact or interview the relatives of hospital patients. I was able to obtain some insight into the relatives' views from letters they had sent to the hospital. In one letter Denise's brother put the family point of view. He denied that Denise was a problem at home and by implication held the care staff responsible:

> After the death of her mother the family
> were unable to look after her permanently
> for various domestic reasons, but we have
> always had her home for weekends. Here
> she is well behaved and helpful and we
> are able to take her out in any company.
> But we gather there are behaviour problems
> while she is at the hostel and it is our
> desire to help in any way we can to over-
> come these, so that she can be happily
> settled.

He did concede that Denise's diabetes could be

195

partly responsible.

> Being diabetic could perhaps account for
> some of the problems, although throughout
> the many years that she has had this
> condition she has appeared to accept it
> very well.

The Traditional Medical View The traditional
medical view placed great emphasis on Denise's
diabetes. Denise's difficult behaviour was
attributed mainly to her diabetes. At a case
conference one consultant stated that "a lot of
Denise's behaviour is due to her low blood sugar
level and one has to make allowances for it". This
consultant also discounted Denise's talk.

> It is easy to over-estimate Denise's
> intelligence on initial meeting, because
> when you first talk to her she seems to be
> telling you very sensible things. However
> if you stay to listen you find it rapidly
> becomes nonsense and does not mean
> anything.

In the traditional medical view, Denise's
relatives were partly responsible for the
problems. Their behaviour had exacerbated Denise's
behaviour problems.

> When Denise's mother died Denise was passed
> from pillar to post. Denise developed a
> lot of attention seeking behaviour during
> this period and staff must try to gratify
> this.

The solution was to disregard Denise's
accusations, to control Denise's diabetes and
minimise the impact of Denise's relatives.

The Progressive Medical View This was almost
the complete opposite of the traditional medical
view. The impact of Denise's diabetes was
minimised, Denise's statements were accepted at
face value and the relatives' expertise
acknowledged. Another consultant's acceptance of
Denise's statements is clear in the following
extract:

> It is quite obvious when one talks to

Denise that she is, in fact, suffering
from what is really a delayed grief
reaction following on the death of her
mother over a year ago. As frequently
happens with low grade patients, it is
only just dawning on her what has
happened ... I think she really summed
up her problem herself when she said to
me "my mother would not let me come here
to start with. What I want is someone
to love me."

This consultant's solution involved
acceptance of the relatives' expertise and special
treatment for Denise within the local authority
hostel to help Denise get over her feelings of
grief.

I explained to the hostel staff that in my
opinion all this girl requires is
virtually individual attention from the
staff during the next few months to tide
her over this reaction.

When this consultant admitted Denise to his own
unit, his attitude changed to the traditional
medical view.

The Clinical Psychologist's View   Denise was
assessed by a clinical psychologist at the
hospital. This psychologist was interested in
Denise's accusations and devoted most of her
report to evaluating them.

At first sight Denise seemed like a rather
well organised girl because her
manner of speaking and moving gives the
impression of decisiveness, and her care
of her person and belongings seems
orderly. It was however, noticeable,
even in a short interview, that she
contradicts herself frequently and picks
up and uses another idea rapidly.
There is no evidence that her
comprehension and reasoning ability is
ever above that of a four or four and a
half year old. When drawing, her
organisation is peculiar. As examples
having drawn what appeared to be a face
and named the eyes, nose and mouth, she

then drew a small circle inside the bigger
one, to one side of the mouth and called
it the "face". As each idea occurred she
just stuck it in somewhere without
hesitation. In view of these findings,
one would be less inclined to see her
"lying" as deliberate alterations of a
given state than as one indication of her
lack of realistic framework into which to
fit her experiences. Memory is always
reconstructive, and she cannot "construct"
properly even in the present.

This view offered something to everybody. It
supported the nurses' view that Denise did not
tell the truth. However it exonerated Denise, she
was not lying. Although Denise was exonerated,
her relatives were not.

Most individuals of her general level of
ability do not confabulate as she does.
Perhaps she has been "expected" by others
to respond in a way beyond her ability?
During the past few years anyway, she has
not had a stable home background with
satisfactory human relationships that
might have provided the needed framework.
And she has been faced with the
necessity of adjusting in one place after
another with family members who say she
is "no trouble" but still cannot offer
her a home so that one wonders if all
the "unreality" is in her. Certainly at
present she is seeking attention and
affection by whatever means she can get
it.

Although the clinical psychologist did not
prescribe a detailed solution, she legitimated the
existing situation. Denise needed stability,
therefore she should stay at the Jane Eagle
Hospital.

The Social Worker's View   The social worker
adopted a psycho-social perspective. Denise's
behaviour was caused by the social situation which
developed after her mother's death. This approach
involved accepting Denise's statements as
statements made by an individual with ability but
it did not involve accepting either Denise's

statements or those made by her relatives at face value. The social worker stated her position at a case conference and maintained it in the face of the traditional medical view.

> Social Worker - I think Denise's behaviour is caused by instability that resulted from her mother's death. Denise was passed round the family. She learnt manipulative behaviour and played off the various groups of the family against each other.

> Consultant - I am a bit surprised. I didn't think Denise was bright enough to manipulate people.

> Social Worker - She definitely does and the statements by the family that Denise is no trouble at home shouldn't be taken at face value. They are a defensive mechanism, that the family uses to present a united front to the world.

Like the clinical psychologist, the social worker did not prescribe a detailed solution, but sought to legitimate the existing situation. Denise needed a stable social situation, therefore she should stay at the Jane Eagle Hospital.

The Nurses' View Despite the traditional medical view of Denise's fragile diabetes and the views of the progressive doctor, psychologist and social worker that Denise was not responsible for her behaviour, the nurses adopted a moral view of Denise. Denise deliberately created problems.

> Looked as if she was having a fit ... although it seemed she was doing this on purpose. Refused breakfast and glucose drink.

In this view Denise was a stable diabetic. Her hypoglycaemic attacks were either simulated or self induced. An extreme version of this view is evident in the following interview with a senior ward nurse:

> Question - What about Denise's attacks?

> Answer - She simulates them for attention
> and to get out of O.T. She doesn't
> expressly dislike O.T., but she goes to
> O.T. because everyone does, she's so
> cantankerous that she feels she won't go
> there ...

> Question - If she's pretending (to have
> attacks) how do you stop her?

> Answer - Give her a big push and see what
> the reaction is. Sometimes I'll turn
> her out of a chair or off her bed and
> watch her when she hits the floor to
> see what her reaction is. Sometimes
> I get a sterile needle and give her a
> poke with it. See if she reacts to it.
> Sometimes she reacts like lightning and
> runs away, sometimes she doesn't.

This nurse interpreted Denise's accusations
as the deliberate lies of a troublemaker not the
product of an incompetent individual. The same
interpretation was applied to the relatives. They
were troublemakers and Denise's defects were the
results of their defects.

> She's basically a warped personality and
> this goes in line with the family history,
> they're all warped personalities.
> They deliberately cause trouble.

As the problems were caused by moral
defect, the solution was moral correction or
punishment. Since punishment was not officially
sanctioned at the Jane Eagle Hospital, it was
never explicitly articulated as a mode of
treatment. However there were occasional
references to it.

> When Denise played up at O.T. we stopped
> her going but she treated this as a
> reward rather than a punishment. She
> was only too happy to stay on the ward.

Since Denise's relatives were seen as a
problem, a major concern was to reduce their
influence. Some nurses advocated discharging
her to relatives' care, this would not only
solve the problem for the hospital, it would also

serve as a punishment for the relatives.

> I'd like to strangle them (her relatives).
> One day they'll pick on the wrong
> consultant and he'll discharge her.
> Dr. T. has been very close to discharging
> her ... After she's discharged it will
> be very difficult to get her in anywhere
> else. Hard to comment on any future.
> It depends on the relatives ... I don't
> know what she could do if we eliminated
> the relatives.

<u>Summary of Views</u> Although all participants agreed there was a problem, their explanations and solutions differed. If we focus on attitudes to Denise's statements then the participants' views can be divided into two main clusters. The relatives and the progressive consultant were prepared to accept Denise's statements. The other views all discounted Denise's views. Nurses sometimes were inconsistent. Some nurses were willing to believe Denise's statements when they threw bad light on the relatives but unwilling to believe them when they threw bad light on the hospital staff.

<u>Denise's Care</u>
As Denise's relatives' and Denise's statements could be discounted by the nurses, they did not create any ideological problems. There was no need to justify Denise's care. Furthermore Denise's diabetes could be used to justify the routine. She had to eat meals not because the staff wanted her to but because it was good for her. However there were still practical problems and these problems were solved in a practical way, i.e. by avoidance where possible and physical control where necessary.

<u>Relationship between Denise's relatives and the</u> <u>hospital staff</u> It would be more accurate to describe this as a nonrelationship. Initially Denise's relatives visited regularly. Each weekend they either visited her or collected her for weekend leave. After they obtained transport for Denise's home visit, the relatives stopped visiting.
The ward staff did not put any obstacles in the way, even though some of them would have liked

to. A policy of non-cooperation was initiated by the ward consultant at Denise's case conference.

> I want it clearly understood that nobody at this end is to make arrangements for transport. No one is to order or to cancel the transport. This is to be left totally to the other end. It is not hospital policy to provide transport for weekend leave. I have requested from Denise's brother a written arrangement outlining which family Denise is going home to each weekend but he has failed to provide this. As far as the hospital is concerned we have absolutely no responsibility for the arrangements. All the arrangements are to be made from the other end.

Relationship between ward staff and Denise   Again the relationship was based on avoidance. Denise spent most of her leisure time sitting on her bed in the dormitory, dozing or looking at magazines. The only contact between ward staff and Denise was during meal times and then it was minimal and functional. At O.T. Denise also spent most of her time sitting in a chair dozing. Little attempt was made to involve Denise in group activities.

Table 8.1 summarises Denise's activities for one Sunday. The avoidance and lack of contact between Denise and the ward staff is clear. Denise spent 6 of the 14 hours in the dormitory sitting on her bed. The ward staff initiated contact with Denise when it was absolutely necessary - at meal times and for her treatment. Even then they attempted to use other patients as intermediaries. On the one occasion Denise sought contact with the nurses, she wanted to help make ward decorations, she was rebuffed. In contrast when Denise sought contact with the other patients, e.g. with two patients who were doing a jigsaw, she was accepted. Generally Denise did not seek help from either the patients or staff on the ward. For example Seagull patients usually went to the hospital canteen after lunch on Sunday. The majority of the patients got ready and went out as a group. Denise avoided the other patients and went by herself. When she returned she showed her purchases to me, the outsider on the ward.

The observations also indicate when avoidance was not possible the relationship tended to become one of tension which often resulted in conflict.

Summary The relationship between Denise's relatives and the hospital staff and between Denise and the ward staff can be best classified as an avoidance relationship. The different groups related to each other only when it was absolutely unavoidable and then the relationships tended to be difficult and full of conflict.

Conclusion
Denise created problems for the staff at the Jane Eagle Hospital, especially for nurses on Seagull Ward. She asserted her individuality by refusing to follow the ward routine and she challenged the competence of the nurses with her accusations of cruelty. Similarly her relatives refused to accept a passive role and were assertive about their own and Denise's rights.

Although Denise could talk about her situation, her accusations did not create a problem of legitimacy. They could be disregarded by the nurses. The emphasis was on practical measures of control, avoidance when possible and control when necessary. Underlying the diversity of opinions expressed by hospital staff was a unifying theme. The statements made by Denise and her relatives could and should be discounted. Although the ward nurses had to carry out the practical measures of control, they could feel they were doing the right thing.

One important aspect of control was the silence about alternatives. In Denise's case we can glimpse one of these silent and suppressed options. In legitimating the existing situation some participants stressed the need for stability. This perhaps was clearest in the social worker's view. The social worker suggested that a large number of people had cared for Denise and this was the cause of Denise's manipulative behaviour. This view had two implications; Denise should stay at the Jane Eagle and her contact with her relatives be reduced; and the number of members of staff caring for Denise should be reduced. Although the first implication was recognised and accepted, the second was not. Using ward records I estimated that 123 different nurses were involved in

Control Strategies

Table 8.1 A Summary of Denise's activities for one Sunday

Time	Activity	Associated Interactions
7.00	Lying in bed awake.	7.05 Complaining that she doesn't like it here.
	Dresses and has insulin.	
8.00	Sitting on bed in dormitory.	8.55 Patient sent to fetch Denise from the dormitory, returns and tells nurse that Denise won't come. Nurse says
9.00	Breakfast.	leave her she'll come.
		9.00 Patient says Denise hasn't come. Nurse fetches Denise.
10.00		
	Sitting on bed in dormitory.	
11.00		
	Cup of tea in kitchen.	
12.00	Lunch.	
	Wandering around dayroom.	
1.00		1.00 Sits on table watching nurses and other patients making ward decorations, not invited
	Watches decorations being made.	to participate, rebuffed when she indicates she wants to help.
	Prepares to go to canteen.	
2.00		2.00 Gets herself ready for visit to canteen and leaves by herself.
	At the canteen.	
3.00	Returns to ward.	3.00 Shows me her purchases when she returns from the canteen.
		3.30 Called by a patient for her milk.

204

Time	Activity	Associated Interactions
4.00	Has drink of milk in the kitchen.	
	Sitting on bed in the dormitory.	4.45 Patient sent to fetch Denise. She does not come. Nurse fetches her.
5.00	Tea.	
	Standing in corridor.	5.45 Nurse locks all outside. doors and sends Denise into the dayroom.
6.00	Watches two patients doing puzzle and then joins in.	
7.00		7.30 Denise sits at table with her supper in front of her but does not eat it. Patient tells nurse and nurse prepares a sandwich for Denise,
8.00	Bed.	which she eats.

Denise's care on Seagull during a 76 week period. All the practical measures adopted were aimed at creating change in Denise not within the institution.

8.3 ALISON

Introduction

In some respects Alison's case was similar to Denise's. The problems were rather similar, periods of difficult behaviour in which she refused to follow the ward routine which were associated with a physical or health problem. The explanations were also similar. However in two important respects Alison was different. She was more able and she was not a recent admission.

Alison's linguistic skills were similar to Denise's but she also had a good memory. For example she memorised details of the family life of nurses and bought their children little presents. She could also talk coherently about her own background and her current situation in hospital.

Alison and Denise were approximately the same age but, while Denise had spent most of her life at home, Alison had spent most of her life in institutional care. Her problems did not have the same novelty or interest as Alison's. The problems, explanations and strategies of control were all well established. I shall examine the problems first, then the explanations and finally the strategies of control.

Problems at the Jane Eagle Hospital

When Alison was first admitted to the Jane Eagle Hospital, she came with a history of cyclical vomiting associated with sullen withdrawn and uncooperative behaviour. At first Alison settled in well and the ward charge nurse wrote the following note:

> Remains content and happy, possibly
> because she is "Top Dog" of the Ward.

However within a week of this note, he added the following note.

> (Spoke too soon!) Not well today.
> Vomited twice. Very withdrawn.

Following this incident Alison had frequent episodes of vomiting and withdrawn behaviour, sometimes together and sometimes separated. In the year I was working on Seagull Ward there was not a single month without an episode of vomiting or withdrawn behaviour.

Alison was capable of talking about her disturbed behaviour. For example I talked to her after one incident in which she ran away to the local general hospital and recorded the following conversation.

> Question - Why did you run away the
> other day?

Answer - I don't know. I felt fed up.

Question - Did you want to go back to the
    General Hospital?

Answer - Yes.

Question - Does anything ever get on your
    nerves on the ward?

Answer - Yes.

Question - What?

Answer - You can't go and do nothing.

Alison could also talk about the deprivations
of hospital life, especially the absence of
contact with her family. One nurse described her
ability in the following way:

Alison is conscious of the fact that she
is in hospital and that she is separated
from her family. When depressed she says
that she would like to get away either
with her married sister or another sister
in a special hospital .... Alison is
acutely conscious of the lack of interest
shown by her family .... Alison goes
through periods of hating her family when
they neglect her and loving them when they
write and has no real concept of them.

Alison's case did not attract a great deal of
discussion. The explanations were already well
established. I could find no clear cut divisions
of opinions.

Explanations of Alison's behaviour

Nurses devoted little energy to explaining
Alison's behaviour. During crisis periods, they
acted rather than talked. Indeed Alison's
problems were so well established that some nurses
felt that little could be gained from discussing
them. However, there was some discussion of three
possible causes; Alison's family, Alison's
physical condition and Alison's personality.
Unlike the discussions of the causes of Denise's
behaviour there was no clear cut relationship
between participants and explanations. I shall
207

therefore organise my discussion into the themes of her family, her physical illness and her position on the ward.

Alison's family Alison came from a deprived background. At the time of her original admission to a mental subnormality hospital, the consultant described her background in the following way:

> Parents both of low intelligence. Failed to maintain children. Parents now separated. Alison is the fourth of five children. The eldest girl has been a patient in a psychiatric hospital. The second girl was at (a mental subnormality hospital) and is now at a Special Hospital. The third girl also attends an E.S.N. school and the youngest boy is severely subnormal and on the local authority waiting list for hospital care. It is clear, therefore, that the genetic loading is unsatisfactory.

This consultant associated Alison's contemporary problems with her family background.

> Alison's behaviour difficulties and bouts of severe vomiting date at least from the break up of the home.

Alison's mother did try to re-establish contact with Alison but the contact was officially discouraged and she made no further attempts.
When questioned about Alison's difficult behaviour, nurses suggested it could be caused by her relationship with her family.

> Question - What do you think is the cause of Alison's disturbed behaviour?

> Answer - I don't really know except possibly loss of family. No contact with any of her family. When she gets badly withdrawn, that's about the one thing she'll talk about or complain about, that her sisters don't write and that she doesn't see her mum. Mainly that her sisters don't write.

Alison's physical illness During some of her

withdrawn periods Alison also complained of
stomach pains and vomited. Attitudes to Alison's
physical condition varied, both between staff and
over time. When Alison was first admitted to the
Jane Eagle, despite signs of internal bleeding,
her vomiting was treated as a symptom not a cause
of her behaviour, as in the following record:

> Alison has been complaining of pain in her
> (L) side at times over past week, as these
> attacks disappear when outings are due,
> put down to attention seeking.

A new medical officer on Seagull Ward took
Alison's complaints seriously and arranged for an
investigation at the local general hospital. The
results indicated that there was a physical cause
of her vomiting and that she had a malformed and
inflamed oesophagus:

> Barium meal showed gross oesophageal reflux
> with oesophagitis and stricture formation
> at lower end of oesophagus.

However even after this investigation and
diagnosis some nurses still maintained that Alison
fabricated some of the symptoms.

> Very sullen at times, vomits quite
> frequently, sometimes puts the sickness
> on if she thinks she will get a day off
> from A.T.C. (Adult Training Centre).

Alison's position on the ward Some members of the
staff believed that Alison deliberately induced
vomiting and was deliberately difficult. They
suggested that she did this to maintain a dominant
position on the ward. This desire to maintain a
dominant position is described in the following
O.T. Report:

> Alison can work very well. She picks
> up instructions quickly and is capable
> of carrying them out though she likes the
> attention of supervision ... She is very
> obviously aware that she is better than
> most of the group and sometimes flaunts
> this fact in front of them. She sucks up
> to the staff most of the time and is aware
> of the impression she is making.

During her disturbed periods Alison occasionally attacked other able girls who threatened her dominant position on Seagull Ward. Her attitude towards one such patient was described in the following way:

> Alison was extremely pleased that her "friend" Glynis was being admitted from Great Homefarm Hospital ... However, after Glynis' admission Alison quickly lost interest in her even to the point of animosity as she found her own position on the ward as "top dog" threatened by somebody as able as herself.

No reason If pressed most nurses could suggest reasons for Alison's difficult behaviour, family, physical illness or social situation on the ward. Some nurses took some interest in explaining Alison's behaviour but in most instances it seemed to be a fairly vague interest. Although these nurses could mention and discuss the causes of Alison's behaviour, I felt that they did not attach a great deal of importance to these explanations and that they felt that there was no real reason. In several incidents recorded in the notes, nurses stressed that there was no apparent reason for Alison's behaviour. Members of staff, who argued that there was no real reason for Alison's behaviour tended to play down her intelligence and insight and tended to discount her statements about the causes of her behaviour as in the following case history:

> This girl ... has a tendency to make herself vomit by putting her finger down her throat ... She is said to be emotionally immature, lacks understanding and insight into her needs and is withdrawn and uncooperative at times. These bouts of withdrawal, uncooperative behaviour and monosyllabic speech are often associated with the patient standing still and staring into space or sitting on the floor and may persist for several hours or several days. There is no known precipitating cause ...

Discussion Nurses and other members of staff

offered three main explanations for Alison's
behaviour; her family; her illness; and her
position on the ward. There seemed to be a common
stock of explanations, derived from Alison's own
statements, that nurses could draw on. Nurses who
suggested that there was no real reason also
tended to discount Alison's statements.

The relationship between Alison and the nurses on Seagull Ward

The relationship between Alison and the
nurses was dominated by Alison's behaviour. Her
difficult behaviour affected relationships not
only when she was difficult but also at other
times. I shall first discuss the relationship
during disturbed periods.

The relationship during disturbed periods   When
Alison was disturbed, nurses responded by
isolating her and using drugs to control her
behaviour. The response of the staff to ten
episodes is summarised in Table 8.2.

The last of these episodes took place while I
was doing fieldwork on Seagull Ward and I recorded
the actions of nurses on one Sunday during the
episode. The following extracts are taken from my
field notes and illustrate the relationship
between Alison and the nurses during this
episode.

Sunday 10.15 Seagull Ward

> K.D. (duty nursing officer) phones ward to
> say Alison is at the General Hospital.
> Alison is reported as violent and hitting
> out. K.D. will come down and get K.T.
> (nurse in charge) and they will fetch
> Alison in K.D.'s car. The nurse in charge
> prepares an injection of Largactil
> (tranquillising drug).

> K.T. - We'll probably need it.

> Andy - Is Alison written up for it?

> K.T. - Probably not, last night's dose was
> probably the only one she was written up
> for.
> K.T. draws 100 mg of Largactil into
> the syringe.

Table 8.2 Ten major episodes of difficult behaviour (extracted from ward records)

Date	Type of Behaviour	Staff Action	Recorded Causes of Difficult Behaviour
May 1971	1. Left ward without permission. 2. Refused to dress. 3. Aggressive to staff.	1. Forcibly returned to ward. 2. Placed in single room. 3. Injection of tranquilliser drug.	1. Alison slapped by a patient. 2. Possibly constipated.
Sept 1971	1. Aggressive to staff. 2. Attacked a patient. 3. Refused medication. 4. Noisy and disruptive.	1. Placed in single room. 2. Injection of tranquilliser drug. 3. Drugs changed.	(None recorded.)
March 1972	1. Aggressive to staff and patients. 2. Broke a window. 3. Refused meals and drugs. 4. Ran away.	1. Placed in single room. 2. Injection of tranquilliser drug. 3. Drugs changed.	1. Alison's sister visited. 2. Vomiting?
May 1972	1. Aggressive to staff and patients. 2. Broke single room door.	1. Placed in single room. 2. Injection of tranquilliser drug. 3. Injection of sedative drug. 4. Drugs changed.	(None recorded)

Control Strategies

Date	Type of Behaviour	Staff Action	Recorded Causes of Difficult Behaviour
July 1972	1. Ran away	(None recorded)	(None recorded)
March 1973	1. Aggressive	1. Forcibly returned to ward	1. Reprimanded for behaviour
	2. Refused to return to ward	2. Placed in single room	
	3. Aggressive behaviour outside nurse training school	3. Injection of tranquilliser drug	
		4. Drugs changed	
May 1973	1. Refused to dress	1. Forcibly returned to ward	1. Premenstrual phase?
	2. Undressed outside administrative block	2. Placed in single room	
June 1974	1. Difficult behaviour outside nurse training school	(None recorded)	1. Notes stressed that there was no reason
Sept 1974	1. Refused to return to ward	1. Forcibly returned to ward	1. Alison's brother on Magpie Ward was also withdrawn
	2. Difficult behaviour outside administrative block	2. Injection of tranquilliser drug	2. Vomiting?

Date	Type of Behaviour	Staff Action	Recorded Causes of Difficult Behaviour
Sept 1974 (cont.)	3. Ran away to the grounds of the psychiatric hospital		
Nov 1974	1. Aggressive to staff and patients	1. Forcibly returned to ward	1. Returned for treatment at at local general hospital
	2. Ran away to the local general hospital	2. Injection of tranquilliser drug	2. Associated with vomiting
	3. A nuisance at the administrative block		

10.20 Seagull Ward

K.T. (to patient Sarah). Will you please clear out your side room. We may need it.
(Patient Sarah takes all the furniture out except the bed.)

10.30 Seagull Ward

K.D. (duty nursing officer) arrives on ward. Telephones duty consultant at home. Explains patient Alison has absconded and is at General Hospital. Stresses patient is violent and requests an injection of Largactil.

Duty consultant agrees, prescribes

100 mg of Largactil three times a
day to be given by injection if the
patient will not take it orally.

K.D. requests a male member of staff in
case Alison is difficult. I offer
to go.   Duty consultant agrees.

10.35 - 10.45 Drive to the General Hospital

K.D. - It's lucky that it was Dr. T. Some
of them aren't so understanding. Mind
you, you still have to tell T.   It's no
good asking for an injection, you have
to tell them to prescribe one. It's a
good job Dr. T.'s O.K.

K.T. - We'll probably have real trouble with
Alison. I can't handle her when she gets
really bad. She can be really violent and
aggressive. I was on the ward on my own
once when Alison "went up the stick"
(i.e. was disturbed). She stood on the
ledge in the six bedded dormitory throwing
tins and everything at me. I got out of
the way and let her get on with it.

K.D. - We're in a really difficult position
because Alison is an informal patient.
Dr. T. said we've got to be careful.
We've got to ask her if she wants to come
back before we wade in.

K.T. - There's no point in doing that
because it'll just give her time to start
hitting out and then we'll have real
problems with her. We might as well get
stuck in straight away.

Andy - Can we bring her back forcibly if
she's a danger to herself or to others?

K.D. - She's an informal patient. We have
no right to bring her back forcibly. We
should really get a social worker to put
her on a section (of the 1959 Mental
Health Act) before we force her to come
back.

10.45 General Hospital, Outpatients Department

K.T. goes in and comes out. Alison is in
the Department. We all go in. Alison
is sitting quietly on one of the benches
next to the entrance. Two porters from
the General Hospital are standing with
her. She has her face in her hands. I
sit next to her. K.D. stands by her and
K.T. stands next to the entrance with the
syringe of Largactil behind her back.

Andy - Will you come back with us?

Alison (Shakes her head. Then to K.D.) -
Yes, I'll go with you.
(Clings to K.D.)

(K.D. leads Alison to the car and she gets
in.)

10.45 - 10.55 Drive back to Jane Eagle Hospital

K.T. - I was really surprised when I went
into the Outpatients. I expected Alison
to start throwing things at me when she
saw me. I was ready to put my head down
and dive for it. All I saw at first were
the two porters. I asked them if they had
one of our patients and I couldn't believe
it when they pointed to Alison sitting
quietly on the chair. I couldn't believe
it when she came out so quickly. She
didn't even need an injection.

10.55 Seagull Ward

(Alison will only get out with K.D. She
puts her arms round K.D.'s neck and K.D.
leads her into the ward and puts her into
bed. All the staff gather in the nurses'
office.)

K.D. - We'll have to give Alison her
injection. We need a few more over to
hold Alison down. She'll really fight
when she sees the injection.

K.T. - Nurse M. is on Pelican but he's no
good.

K.D. phones up B. (charge nurse on Beaver)

216

and asks him to come over with J. (a male
nursing assistant).

11.05   Dormitory of Seagull Ward

(Alison is given an injection. B. and J.
hold her arms. I hold her legs.
K.T. gives the injection. Alison goes
to sleep.)

The relationship at other times   Alison's
disturbed behaviour affected her relationship with
the nurses in various other ways. Alison was
given a relatively privileged position on Seagull
Ward. Her privileges were an acknowledgement of
her abilities but they were also a concession to
her disruptive potential. One nurse described her
treatment in the following way:

Although she is bright and friendly she
is extremely repetitive and after an
initial period of friendliness it becomes
hard not to get irritated by her.
Because of Alison's frequent periods of
disturbed behaviour it is important not
to convey this feeling of irritation in
case it precipitates an outburst, and one
therefore tends to have far more patience
with her than with other patients.

When Alison was first admitted a scheme was
devised for increasing her contact with her
family. Her brother, David, was living on Magpie
Ward and an attempt was made to foster a
relationship between the two siblings. A strategy
was devised at a case conference after Alison's
admission and recorded in the conference report:

It was reported that although Alison is
much more intelligent than her brother
David ... and despite the fact that she
did not recognise him on arrival she
enjoys helping him and he has responded
well to her interest.
The question of eventual placement outside
hospital was discussed. It was felt that
any plans made should be such that they
might suit David as well. As a pair they
could offer each other mutual support -
and Alison could help David practically.

> The possibility of increasing the
> opportunities for brother and sister to be
> together was raised. It should be
> possible, for instance, for Alison to go
> shopping in the village with David.

This attempt to increase the contact between
Alison and her family, within the framework of the
hospital, was rejected by Alison.   One nurse
described Alison's attitude to her brother in the
following way:

> Her brother David is on Magpie Ward but
> Alison is rather ashamed of him and
> thinks he is dim.

At a subsequent case conference the strategy was
abandoned.

<u>Discussion</u>   The relationship between Alison and
the nurses on Seagull Ward took place within the
framework of the hospital.   Alison could be
indulged as long as she did not challenge the
basic order within the hospital.   When she was
disturbed staff reacted with measures designed to
maintain order within the ward. When she was not
disturbed staff acted on those of her complaints
that could be satisfied within the existing order
of the hospital. Solutions outside this framework
were not considered.   One nurse did discuss a
solution outside this framework but discounted
it.

> Nursing staff ... are more tolerant
> towards her in the hope she will behave
> well. In my case, it was not solely
> with this object in mind that I showed
> a degree of tolerance that I wouldn't
> otherwise have done, but in the back
> of my mind I always felt that Alison's
> future was so empty. She was a bright
> girl with a fair amount of insight and
> her past, present and future are in
> hospital ... Her behaviour precludes her
> from any existence in the community but
> one cannot help considering how much her
> background caused her mental condition.
> I always felt that she must suffer
> considerably from regular staff changes
> as it gave her no opportunity to form a

stable and permanent relationship with anybody. Alison is badly lacking a close relationship with anyone but even if this were possible in a staff/patient situation it is questionable whether or not she is capable of forming one.

Conclusion

Alison, like Denise, presented the ward staff with multiple problems. Not only was she occasionally withdrawn and sullen, and physically ill but she could also discuss her situation with,according to some nurses, insight. There appeared to be in her case a stock of explanations - family background, physical illness and relations on the ward - that nurses could draw on if they wanted. Some nurses used these explanations with conviction, others did not. However when Alison was difficult all the nurses tended to react directly to the difficult behaviour rather than to the possible underlying causes.

Alison's disturbed behaviour dominated her relationship with the staff. While she was difficult she was subject to physical control. When she was "well" she was indulged. Although this indulgence had a practical objective, i.e. to prevent a deterioration of her behaviour, nurses could justify it by reference to Alison's obvious ability. Strategies were proposed that related to the explanation for Alison's behaviour, i.e. attempts were made to foster a relationship between Alison and her brother, but these strategies were limited to the existing framework of the hospital. Strategies that involved changing this framework were discounted as impractical.

8.4 EVA

Introduction

Eva was one of the most able patients in the hospital. Nurses could not deny Eva's competence. She had led an independent life in the community. She had been married and had a son, although he was now in care. The practical problems presented by Eva were probably less difficult than those presented by Alison or Denise. Although she could be uncooperative and even violent, this was only after considerable provocation. The problems she presented were mainly those of legitimacy. With the evidence of former independence how could the nurses justify her present dependent condition? Eva was resident at the Jane Eagle for two separate periods. As the problems of each stay were different I shall discuss them separately.

Eva's first stay at the Jane Eagle Hospital

In this part I shall examine Eva's background, the initial problems she presented and the initial strategies staff proposed for coping with these backgrounds.

Eva's background Eva was born in 1945. Her mother and two brothers were described in the records as of "low intelligence" and her father was violent towards her. Apart from short periods at a special school for educationally subnormal children, she had had no education. When she was 18, she was admitted to a mental subnormality hospital. However her stay was relatively short. She was allowed to become housekeeper to Mr. D. who was 30 years older than her and who had known her since childhood. In 1964 they married and in 1965 they had a son. Eva was unable to care for her son and he was taken into care by the local authority. When Eva's husband died in 1972, she was admitted to the Jane Eagle Hospital.

Problems at the Jane Eagle Hospital When Eva was first admitted, there were two interrelated problems. What sort of future should Eva have and how would she adjust to the future that was selected for her? The consultant decided that Eva was unable to look after herself but did not need long term hospitalisation. Eventually he planned to discharge her to a local authority hostel.

> Since her husband's death she has not been willing to contemplate giving up her three-bedroomed house, but does not seem to realise that the rent still has to be paid when she is not there. At present the hospital is paying, but the council would like the house partly because Mrs. D.'s relations with some of her neighbours were poor ... It seemed generally agreed that Mrs. D would need considerable help and supervision

> for the present. Some arrangements
> about her furniture and relinquishing her
> home will therefore be necessary ..
> specifically it was suggested that Mrs. F.
> (medical social worker) talk to her, take
> her to select furniture, etc., and get in
> touch with the Housing Authority.

Much to the surprise of the ward nurses, Eva
was persuaded, without too much pressure, to give
up her house and store her furniture and even went
to her house to select furniture. However, the
decision had repercussions. Eva's behaviour
deteriorated soon afterwards. About two weeks
after she agreed to give up her house the
following nursing note was made.

> Uncooperative behaviour. Refused to help
> on ward and also refuses her daily bath.
> Wanders away from ward.

Nurses felt uneasy about the decision about
Eva's future and cooperated with the ward
consultant in developing a therapy programme for
Eva.

Therapy Programme: A Strategy of Legitimation
Staff acknowledged that Eva had potential for
independence and a therapy programme was initiated
to maintain this independence. It involved
improving Eva's physical condition, improving her
personal hygiene, developing her domestic skills
and preparing her for open employment.

Diet. When Eva was admitted, she weighed over 20
stones and this had affected her heart. The
consultant prescribed a reducing diet for her.
Even when she was uncooperative in other ways, Eva
kept to this diet and rapidly lost weight. Within
a year she had lost three and a half stone and two
years after admission she weighed just over 13
stones.

Personal hygiene. Eva's personal hygiene was
poor. Furthermore she had a scalp infection that
was diagnosed as psoriasis. In view of Eva's
obesity and her psoriasis, the consultant
prescribed extra baths for her. Eva was
uncooperative and difficult about bathing. One
nurse described one incident as follows:

221

> It was when Eva first came in. I asked her
> if she wanted a bath but she refused. It
> was rare in those days for her to have a
> bath. As far as I was concerned she could
> stink. S. (duty nursing officer) came
> round and asked me if I had any problems.
> I said none except Eva would not have a
> bath. He said "We'll see about that.
> I'll get her in the bath. I've already
> done it a couple of times. If she won't
> go in, I'll put her in clothes and all!"
> So he went off down the "backs" (toilets,
> bathroom etc.). After a bit, we thought
> S. had been gone for quite a long time, so
> I went down the "backs". I found him
> lying on his back with Eva standing over
> him. He wasn't unconscious, he was just
> dazed. He got up as I came in. I asked
> him if he was alright, he said yes. Then
> I ran over to Leopard and told B.
> (charge nurse) that we were having trouble
> on Seagull and would he come over and give
> a hand. B. did and they got Eva in the
> bath and bathed her.

Domestic skills. Eva was to develop domestic skills on the ward to prepare for more independent life. She was to help at mealtimes, by handing out meals, pouring tea etc. She was to look after her own clothes, especially wash and repair her own underwear.

Initially Eva was rather uncooperative and after the decision to give up her house she totally refused help.

> Eva still refuses to go to O.T. All she
> does is sit in her chair all day. If you
> ask her to do something then you get told
> "I'm tired" or "No, I don't want to".

Training for Open Employment. The consultant asked the Occupational Therapy Unit to teach Eva to use a sewing machine. The failure of the scheme was recorded in the following way.

> Eva was referred to the department (O.T.)
> to be taught to use the sewing machine.
> It was felt that she might progress to
> the necessary standards which are needed
> to obtain a job as a seamstress, in open

> employment ... Eva's main problem was
> that she leaned heavily on the material
> and thus hampered its progress through
> the machine. She was very slow and
> cautious and stopped for many rests ...
> I have much doubt that Eva will ever make
> the grade as a seamstress and also
> because her heart really isn't in it. A
> job involving mainly hand sewing in a
> "sheltered" sewing room, which does not
> have the pressures of open employment
> seems a more realistic possibility.

Failure of the therapy programme After nine months
at the Jane Eagle, Eva was transferred to a small
unit for the mentally handicapped. It was
generally accepted that the therapy programme had
failed.

In theory Eva should have been trained for a
more independent life, in practice the need to
control Eva made this impossible. The therapy
programme needed Eva's cooperation but following
the decision to give up her house, she became
difficult. Eva's difficult behaviour was
controlled in the routine way, through drugs.

> Eva is being disturbed the past couple of
> weeks. Wandering off from the hospital
> on a couple of occasions. Bouts of
> crying, refusing to go to O.T. Restart
> Tofranil 25 mg TDS.

The need to control Eva conflicted with the
needs of the therapy programme. For example for
her training as a seamstress Eva had to go to the
O.T. unit but, when she was difficult, it was
easier to keep her on the ward.

> Wandering away from ward. Felt by ward
> staff to be mainly an objection to O.T.
> Suggest giving her ward duties ...

The practical measures of control took precedence
over the therapy programme.

Discussion of the problems and strategies adopted
after Eva's admission Eva presented staff with
both a practical problem and a problem of
legitimacy. In practical terms she was a patient
like any other patient and in practice she was

controlled in the same way. However in her case
it was more difficult to justify this. She was a
widow with a son. There was evidence that she had
been competent and could under the right
circumstances be independent. Eva provoked not so
much a crisis of control as a crisis of
legitimacy. The therapy programme was to
legitimate the situation. The bad conscience of
one nurse was evident in the following account:

> I think we've been tending to ignore
> Eva as if she doesn't exist at times.
> She's been a social embarrassment to us.
> We had to get her to get rid of her house.
> Then we've had the problem of dealing with
> her son and a person who's been married.
> We haven't had it before and it's been
> difficult for us to cope with, because
> we've got so many low grades ...
> If she was taught the basic ways of
> running a house, looking after her own
> washing and feeding herself on an adequate
> diet there's no reason why she shouldn't
> share a house with somebody else ...
> Dr. T. was a damn good doctor who had his
> own ideas what we were going to do with
> this high grade, the first real high grade
> we'd had ...

This nurse was not emphasing the practical
problems of caring for Eva, for example, the
nurses did not actually have to care for Eva's
son, but the intellectual problems. Eva was
clearly different from the other patients and this
nurse used the usual hospital shorthand to
describe this difference.

Eva : Other patients :: High-grade : Low-grade ::
married : unmarried.

Yet in practical terms Eva was treated in just the
same way as the other patients.

Eva's second stay at the Jane Eagle Hospital

Five months after her transfer to the mental
handicap unit, Eva was readmitted to the Jane
Eagle Hospital. Staff at the unit were unable to
control Eva. She had been wandering off. Two
months after her readmission the deputy ward
sister decided to do a pregnancy test on Eva. The

result was positive. In this section I shall examine the different attitudes to Eva's pregnancy and the strategy staff adopted to deal with the pregnancy and Eva's sex life.

Attitudes to Eva's Pregnancy There was an "official" and "unofficial" view of Eva's pregnancy. The official view was put forward by the medical staff and senior nurses including the ward charge nurse. The unofficial view was put forward by junior nurses.

The Official View. Eva was seen as incompetent. She was a resident in the mental handicap hospital and she had been unable to care for her first child. She did not understand what was involved, therefore she should have the pregnancy terminated and should be prevented from having any more pregnancies. The holders of the official view disregarded Eva's statements about the situation. The ward charge nurse described the situation in the following way:

> I talked to Eva about it (her pregnancy) and she said she knew she was pregnant before the test. She was very unrealistic about the whole thing. She said she wanted the baby. I asked her what she would do with it. She said Debby (an elderly patient) would look after it. I explained that that was impossible. She had no other suggestions.

The Unofficial View. Nurses holding this view almost completely reversed the arguments behind the official view. Eva was or had been competent. Her son was evidence of this.

> Eva had been used to a normal life and she did not think it was wrong to go out and find herself another baby, get herself pregnant again. She'd had a normal married life.

Although the nurses holding this view acknowledged the practical problems involved they also felt it was important that Eva should have her baby. The holders of this view stressed the importance of the pregnancy for Eva and accepted her statements about it.

225

Nurse T. - Eva's very depressed about them taking her baby away. Eva's different from all the other girls on Seagull. She's already had a baby before.

Nurse K. - They're creating more problems with Eva.

Nurse T. - Eva's going to be awful if they take her baby away. She's already got depressed and cried on my shoulder. I booked it in the Report Book.

Andy - Are you sure Eva really wants her baby?

Nurse T. - Yes, because she's really depressed. Eva asked me why they were taking her baby. You can see how depressed she is from the way she walks.

Eva's pregnancy The official view prevailed. Its advocates represented legitimate authority in the organisation and could therefore impose their view. The situation was presented as not only practical but also as right, i.e in the best interest of Eva. The ward charge nurse described the decision in the following way:

Question - What about Eva?

Answer - She's pregnant but we've got her to sign forms for an abortion and sterilisation.

Question - How?

Answer - Dr. T. and Dr. F. came down (to the ward). They interviewed her in the Visitors Room. I was present. They told her she was in the club and she said she understood about being pregnant. She said she did not want to keep the baby.

Question - Was any pressure brought to bear on Eva?

Answer - If she had said there and then that she wanted the baby that would have been

the end of it, she would have had the
baby, but she knew who the doctors were,
she knew that they were important and she
knew she had to agree.

Question - Was any pressure put on Eva?

Answer - They started it in a very clever
way and put it to Eva that it was in her
best interest. I was neutral about it.
K. and T. (nurses cited above) had told
Dr. T. that Eva had told them that she
wanted to keep the baby.

Eva's pregnancy was terminated and she was
sterilised at the local general hospital.

Dealing with the consequences Although ward nurses
had to accept the practical solution, they felt
uneasy. They did not feel it was right. They
blamed the doctors and felt that they were left to
deal with a situation created by the doctors.
However, soon after Eva's termination, an
opportunity arose for the nurses to show their
solidarity with Eva, to expose the incompetence
(and impracticality) of the doctors and
reestablish their mastery of the practical
situation.

Charge Nurse S. - The doctors did another
really stupid thing. We managed to book
an extra outing at the last minute. We
only had a week's warning. Eva was
booked to go to the clinic at the General
Hospital the same day to have her
stitches removed. I told F. (ward medical
officer) that I thought the appointment
ought to be cancelled and Eva ought to
go on the outing. Dr. F. had gone to ask
Dr. T. what she (ward consultant) thought
and Dr. T. had insisted that Eva should
keep her appointment. T. wanted me to
take Eva over to Pelican Ward for the day
and then she would go from there. It was
ludicrous ... I wasn't going to take Eva
over to Pelican when the rest of the girls
were getting on a bus for a day out. I
didn't want to fight with her and that's
what I told Dr. F., but she still
insisted. So I phoned up D. (Senior

227

Nursing Officer) and told him that I
wasn't taking Eva over to Pelican ...
D. must have agreed with me because
I didn't hear anything back from him.
I suppose he must have had a word with
Dr. T. about it.

Nurse K. - It was ludicrous wanting to send
Eva over to Pelican. They had enough
problems of their own. They only had
three staff (on duty), they were already
getting three extra patients we couldn't
take and on top of that Joan had died that
morning ... We gee'd up Eva to go on the
bus. She went on and refused to get off.
Dr. F. came down to try to persuade her to
get off and go to Pelican. It made me
laugh because Dr. F. asked Eva if she
would go to the hospital. Eva told her
that she might go to the hospital but
she definitely wouldn't go today.
Nothing that F. said would make her
change her mind. I got out of the way
because at one stage I thought Eva
was going to lash out. She was rubbing
her hands together and banging one fist
against the other. I didn't want to be
in the way.

Andy - Did F. know what danger she was in?

Nurse K. - I'm sure she didn't because she
was leaning right over Eva trying to
persuade her. Eventually she gave up
and asked S. (charge nurse) if he was
prepared to take her. She asked S. how
he knew that Eva would not play up on the
outing and what he would do if she did.
S. said he was prepared to take the risk.
Eva spent the rest of the outing laughing
to herself. When we came out of the pub
on the way back, Eva laughed and said "I
think I'm a bit pissed".

Charge Nurse S. - There are going to be some
problems about getting her to the clinic
next week because the O.T. are having
an outing and they've got her down to go.

Nurse K. - I've already talked to Eva about

it. I asked her if she wanted to go
to the hospital. She said "I don't
know". I told her that she had got us
into awful trouble with the doctors about
not going this time. Eva asked me what
they were going to do to her at the
hospital I told her that they just wanted
to look at her scar to see how it had
healed. She said "In that case I'll go".

Discussion Eva was discharged to a local authority
social services hostel about a year after the
termination of her pregnancy. Her second stay at
the Jane Eagle was dominated a major practical
problem, her pregnancy. Holders of the official
view stressed the impracticality of the situation
and advocated termination. Holders of the
unofficial view, while acknowledging the practical
problems felt that in theory there was another
solution. The practical solution and the doctors
prevailed. To reestablish their control and to
salve their consciences, the nurses allowed, even
encouraged, Eva to flout authority.
    Despite this indulgence nurses still felt
uneasy about Eva's position on the ward and one
nurse summarised the situation in the following
way:

She's not a lot of trouble on the ward, but
when she does give trouble she really can
give it. But then you can't blame her.
Honestly how would you like it, if you had
lived in the community. You'd been
married and had a child and suddenly you
were herded in with 29 other patients that
had never known an outside life, that
don't talk about anything but going to the
club, going to O.T., going to the Adult
Training Centre ...

Question - Do you think she's becoming cut
off from the outside world?

Answer - Yes she's more like a prisoner. I
think we're inclined to pull her down
rather than let her go up a bit.

Conclusion
    Eva's case was exceptional. Marriage and
parenthood are inextricably linked with

independent adult status. The intellectual problems presented by Eva's case were the reverse of those presented by other patients. With the other patients, especially patients on cot and chair and low grade wards, staff had to deal with humans who had few of the attributes of other humans. In Eva's case they had to deal with a person classified as a dependant, because of her residence in a mental handicap hospital, who had all the attributes of an independent adult. This contradiction was never resolved. There was evidence of incompetence that could be cited, e.g. Eva's son was in care, but this did not supply a satisfactory justification for Eva's position.

Even though nurses felt uneasy about Eva's position, she was still subject to the same restrictions and means of control as other patients. During her first stay an attempt was made to develop a special programme for Eva. This meant changing the normal organisational practices. This programme was abandoned when it proved inconvenient, i.e. conflicted with the practical measures adopted to control Eva.

8.5 CONCLUSION

In this chapter I have examined the problems created by three high grade patients on one high grade ward, Seagull. All three patients created practical problems. Denise was a diabetic patient who refused to follow the ward routine. Alison had bouts of vomiting and periods when she was withdrawn and sullen. Eva was uncooperative during her first stay and pregnant during her second stay. All three patients also presented an ideological threat to the authority of the hospital staff. Denise made accusations of cruelty and her relatives were critical of the care she received. Alison could discuss her problems - her pain, her family and her restriction in the hospital. Eva's status as a widow and parent were difficult to reconcile with her status as a patient. It was also difficult to deny her the status of parenthood when she already had that status.

Dealing with the practical problems was rather easier in each case than dealing with the ideological problem. The nurses had a number of practical measures they could employ quite easily. The routine of basic activities could be used as a

means of control. Failing this, drugs, physical
force and seclusion could all be used.

Most of these controls were personal control,
i.e. they depended on the relationship
between staff and patients. Although personal
control exists outside institutions, e.g. in the
family, the dominant form of control outside care
organisations is impersonal domination exercised
through impersonal mechanisms such as market
forces. Bourdieu has made the following contrast
between:

> social universes in which relations of
> domination are made, unmade and remade in
> and by the interactions between persons,
> and on the other hand, social formations
> in which, mediated by objective,
> institutionalized mechanisms, such as
> those producing and guaranteeing the
> distribution of "titles" (titles of
> nobility, deeds of possession, academic
> degrees, etc.), relations of domination
> have the opacity and the permanence of
> things and escape the grasp of individual
> consciousness and power. (Bourdieu: 1977,
> p.184)

Bourdieu's analysis helps explain one aspect
of the case studies. In Denise's and Alison's
case study, I suggested that there was one
practical measure hinted at but never adopted. It
was suggested that both patients would benefit
from more stable relations with the nurses. Why
was this measure never openly articulated and why
did nurses move frequently between wards? The
domination exercised at the Jane Eagle was
personal. To justify this domination some
mechanism had to be found for depersonalising it,
otherwise staff could be accused of exploiting the
patients for their own personal interest. The
constant movement of nurses between wards was one
way of depersonalising this personal control.

The ideological problems were more difficult
to cope with. In all three cases there was a
tendency to emphasise the incompetence of the
patients and therefore the unreliability of their
statements. This strategy was most successful in
Denise's case and least successful in Eva's case.
Alison and Eva both aspired to greater
independence and objected to the demands made of

them. It was difficult within the existing
framework of the institution to either satisfy
these demands or deny their legitimacy. In Eva's
case the problems were compounded by her anomalous
position. She did not fit into the main categories
of care and so a special programme had to be
designed for her. In her case the problem could
only be "solved" by transferring her to another
care organisation.

CHAPTER 9
CONCLUSION

9.1 INTRODUCTION

In this conclusion I shall concentrate on the three main themes that have run through this book, the hospital as an institution, the hospital as a culture and the relationship between ideas and actions in the hospital.

9.2 THE HOSPITAL AS AN INSTITUTION

In Chapter One, I used a preliminary definition of institutions as organisations in which one group of individuals, the residents, are dependent on another group, the staff, for some or all of the basic necessities of life such as food and clothing. The relationship between the staff and the residents is based on inequality and personal dependency. Outside institutions, relationships of inequality or personal dependency exist but they are usually based on or disguised as relationships of kinship. Otherwise relationships are, in theory, relationships of equality, contractual relations established between formally independent and equal individuals.

The relationship between the staff and the patients at the Jane Eagle Hospital was indeed one of dependency. There were several ways in which this relationship was maintained, through the patient classification system, through the daily routine of basic care and, when all else failed, through physical control. The classification of patients discussed in Chapters Three to Five was an ideology, it involved specific definitions of reality. The classification was a definition made

by members of the hospital staff, especially
nurses, not definitions made by the patients
themselves or by the patients' relatives. The
definitions of the patients and their relatives
had little impact as neither group had the
resources, organisation and practical mastery of
the situation, to impose their definitions. For
example the medical and nursing staff controlled
the movement of patients between wards and this
was both a cause and effect of the classification,
a cause in so far as patients with similar
characteristics were grouped together and an
effect in terms of the ward allocation of any
individual patient.

The classification of patients was a
definition of reality within the hospital and the
rapid movement of nurses between wards described
in Chapter Six ensured that nurses were
socialised into the hospital culture and accepted
this definition of reality. The routine of basic
care involved practical measures of control. In
Chapter Seven I showed how nurses exercised
control over patients, during mealtimes. This
control was related to the common features of the
organisation of meals on the three wards. There
was no commensality. The staff provided the food,
the patients ate it. The staff decided what was
eaten, and how, where and when it was eaten. The
differences in the organisation of the meals on
the three wards were related to differences in the
problems of control and problems of feeding. The
purpose of meals was to feed the patients. Even
the most able patients in the hospital were
incapable of obtaining their own food and many of
the cot and chair patients could not feed
themselves. In this sense the dependency of the
patients was intrinsic not imposed and the control
exercised during the meals was a necessary means
to the end of providing the patients with
sustenance.

There were aspects of the control exercised
during meal time that could not be explained by
the need to feed the patients. Nurses could use
meals to symbolise and legitimate their control.
Meals formed a central organisational focus and
meal times set the rhythm of the institution. They
created a cyclical group time that structured the
interactions within the hospital.

Some patients rejected the routines and rules
and tried to maintain their own individual time

Conclusion

and their own independent life. In Chapter Eight,
I examined the cases of three high grade patients.
All three rejected the routine and the cyclical
time of the institution and attempted to maintain
their independence. In each case similar measures
of physical control were used. However,in all
three cases the patients talked about their
situation and this created problems of legitimacy.
These could be resolved when the nurses could
discount the patients' statements but remained
more intractable when they could not.

There were at the Jane Eagle Hospital three
modes of control, the ideological control
exercised through the patient classification
system, control exercised through technical
activities and the physical control of individuals
through drugs or isolation. These three modes of
control can be seen as three dimensions of power.
The physical control of individuals conforms to a
common sense definition of power. It is power
visibly, overtly and consciously exercised. This
type of power would fit within traditional
definitions of power such as Tawney's definition
of power as:

> the capacity of an individual, or a group
> of individuals, to modify the conduct of
> other individuals or groups in the manner
> which he desires, and to prevent his own
> being modified in the manner he does not.
> (cited in Smith: 1976, p.16)

However the overt physical control of
individuals is a crude and blunt instrument and
was used at the Jane Eagle Hospital only as a last
resort. The most sophisticated form of power at
the Jane Eagle was the classification of
patients. It was an ideological control of
reality. Ideological control operates by
excluding alternatives. The reality as defined is
not just a reality it is the reality. There is no
alternative. Lukes has defined this form of power
in the following way:

> Is it not the supreme and insidious exercise
> of power to prevent people, to whatever
> degree, from having grievances by shaping
> their perceptions, cognitions and
> preferences in such a way that they accept
> their role in the existing order of

things, either because they can see or
imagine no alternative to it, or because
they see it as natural and unchangeable
or because they value it as divinely
ordained and beneficial. (Lukes: 1974,
p.24)

Whereas physical power is explicit,
consciously exercised and has a direction from
controller to controlled, ideological power is
implicit, unconsciously exercised and pervasive.
It affects those who exercise it as well as those
over whom it is exercised. The classification of
patients is a means by which nurses and other
staff "order", i.e. place in categories, the
patients and this facilitates the staff management
of the patients. However the insidious and
sophisticated affects are produced on the
classifiers and those who apply the classification
rather than on the patients who are classified and
do not know or share the knowledge of the
classification. The classification excludes
alternatives for the classifiers and those who
apply the classification. Bourdieu has referred
to exclusion of alternatives as "doxa" and he
describes the nature of "doxa" and its
consequences in the following way:

Systems of classification which reproduce,
in their own specific logic, the objective
classes, i.e. the divisions of sex, age,
or position in the relations of
production, make their specific
contribution to the reproduction of the
power relations of which they are the
product, by securing the misrecognition
and hence the recognition, of the
arbitrariness on which they are based ...
This experience we shall call doxa, so as
to distinguish it from an orthodox or
heterodox belief implying awareness and
recognition of the possibility of
different or antagonistic beliefs.
(Bourdieu: 1977, p.164)

In my study, I have identified a third form
of power that is neither physical control nor part
of the collective ideology but was closely related
to both. It was evident in the organisation of
meals at the hospital. The provision of food was

an instrumental activity. The patients had to be fed. They were dependent on the nurses for their food. However, this instrumental activity could be used as an additional means of control. Nurses decided how, where and when the patients ate and the patients had to accept these conditions. Each meal demonstrated the nurses' control over the patients. Indeed the distribution of patients' drugs at mealtimes was not only convenient but also symbolically apt. Drugs were a major means of patient control.

Most patients accepted the food on the conditions on which it was offered but some did not. These patients were subject to a variety of pressures, including physical control. Failure to follow the collective routine was not just a cause of control, it was also used to justify this control. The statement "patients had to eat" was read as "patients had to eat on the terms dictated by nurses and other staff". When there were difficulties, nurses always sought change within the patient, never within the institution. Because the alternatives were suppressed and hidden, it was difficult to see them, but in the three case studies presented in Chapter Eight there were occasional glimpses of the suppressed alternatives, the changes that could be made in the institution not in the individual patient. All the patients would have benefited from more stability but the regular movement of nurses was necessary for the maintenance of the structure of the ward classification and the strategies of patient control.

The organisation of meals was also related to the classification of patients and the associated definition of reality. The patients on the three types of wards were seen as having different needs and these needs were used to justify the different organisations of meals on the three wards. However these "needs" did not fully explain the organisation of meals on the different wards. There were on each ward patients whose needs were seen as different to those of other patients, e.g. cot and chair patients on low grade wards were treated differently to the cot and chair patients on cot and chair wards. I did not, as a social scientist, believe that it was my role to evaluate the "objective needs" of the patients. This is essentially a medical or scientific question which the social scientist is not specifically competent

to answer. As a social scientist I was interested
in the "needs" attributed to the patients, why
they were seen as having them and how this
affected social relations.

The control of residents during and through
technical activities, especially in the provision
of the basic necessities of life, was a form of
control that was characteristic of and developed
within the institution. The mental handicap
hospital was a medical institution that cared for
and controlled one type of dependant and one form
of dependency. The medical ideology was important
because it helped to disguise the control within
the ideology of care. The ambiguity I found
between the meal as a way of providing patients
with food and the meal as a means of patient
control permeated the institution. All custodial
control, i.e. guarding and isolating the patients,
could be justified by reference to remedial
medical care, i.e. making the patient better,
preventing suffering etc.. In the routine of
basic care, control could both protect the
patient against accident and mishap and could also
act to correct or even punish the patient. The
three "high grade" patients discussed in Chapter
Seven challenged this ambiguity by forcing a
polarisation and separation between the custodial
and the remedial. The success of the institution
depends on maintaining the ambiguity between care
and control.

The development of medicine as a benign or
humanitarian form of control has been described by
Freidson:

> In our day, what has been called crime,
> lunacy, degeneracy, sin and even poverty
> in the past is now being called illness,
> and social policy has been moving toward
> adopting a perspective appropriate to the
> imputation of illness. Chains have been
> struck off and everywhere health
> professionalism has been raised to
> legitimate the claim that the proper
> management of deviance is "treatment" in
> the hands of a responsible and skilled
> profession. The labels of sin and crime
> being removed, what is done to the deviant
> is likely to be said to be done for his
> own good, done to help him rather than
> punish him, even though the treatment

> itself may constitute a deprivation under
> ordinary circumstances. (Freidson:1975,
> p.213)

Freidson stressed the role of medicine in controlling deviance for and on behalf of society. Freidson derived his definition of deviance from Becker (1963, p.9). Becker proposed a fairly broad definition of deviance as an activity that breaks a social rule or norm. Freidson avoided a discussion of the nature of these rules by examining the effect of rule breaking rather than the causes of rule breaking or the nature of the rules. He justified this emphasis by stressing the neglect by sociologists of the consequences of rule breaking.

> (Sociologists of deviance) have followed
> the model of medicine in setting as their
> task the determination of some stable,
> objective quality or state of deviance
> (e.g. criminal behaviour) and have sought
> to determine its etiology. (Freidson:
> 1975, p.213)

Although I have examined only the internal relations of the hospital in this book, I believe that these relations can throw some light on wider social issues. I have argued that there were three dimensions to the power of the hospital staff, physical control, control through technical activities and ideological control. All three forms of control were expressed in and structured the relations between groups of staff and groups of patients. Despite the depersonalisation of control through the regular movement between wards of nurses described in Chapter Six, this control was exercised in face to face relations. This personalised exercise of control can be seen as a "primitive" and "inefficient" form of control when compared to the impersonal forms of domination exercised outside institutions, e.g. through market forces. It is "primitive" in the sense that it is characteristic of simpler societies (Bourdieu: 1977, pp.183-197). It is "inefficient" in the sense that is requires constant effort by individuals to maintain the status quo. The formal equality of contractual relations conceals domination exercised within and through the market, e.g. labour and capital do not meet as

equals in the market place. The difference
between personalised domination inside the
institution and impersonal domination outside
suggests that, despite their obvious diversity,
institutions perform a common function within our
society. Individuals, who cannot or will not
submit to the impersonal forms of domination
exercised outside institutions, are subject to the
personal forms of domination within them.

9.3 THE HOSPITAL AS A CULTURE

In this book, I have treated the hospital as
a culture. In this section I shall examine the
concept of culture and its applicability to the
Jane Eagle Hospital. Tylor defined culture in the
following way:

> Culture or civilization, taken in its wide
> ethnographic sense, is that complex whole
> which includes knowledge, belief, art,
> morals, law, custom, and any other
> capabilities and habits acquired by man
> as a member of society. (Tylor: 1958,
> p.1)

This all-embracing definition of culture
cannot be applied to the Jane Eagle Hospital if it
is taken to imply culture as some integrated and
isolated whole. Not only was the hospital part of
a wider society and culture, i.e. English society,
but different participants in the hospital were
also members of distinct occupational groups which
had their own distinctive occupational
sub-cultures and values, e.g. doctors and nurses.
However, the idea of a culture as a singular
distinctive integrated whole was a nineteenth
century myth. As Radcliffe-Brown pointed out:

> It is rarely that we find a community that
> is absolutely isolated, having no outside
> contact. At the present moment of
> history, the network of social relations
> spreads over the world, without any
> absolute solution of continuity anywhere.
> (Radcliffe-Brown: 1952, p.193)

Radcliffe-Brown's solution was to adopt a
laissez-faire attitude. The researcher could take
"any convenient locality of a suitable size"

Conclusion

(Radcliffe-Brown: 1952, p.193) as his or her basic
unit. Levi-Strauss followed Radcliffe-Brown
when he defined a single culture as:

> a fragment of humanity which, from the
> point of view of the research at hand and
> the scale on which the latter is carried
> out, presents significant discontinuities
> in relation to the rest of humanity.
> (Levi-Strauss: 1968, p.295)

With Levi-Strauss's pluralistic definition of
culture the designation of the Jane Eagle Hospital
would be no problem as:

> the same set of individuals may be
> considered to be parts of many different
> cultural contexts: universal,
> continental, national, regional, local,
> etc., as well as familial, occupational,
> religous, political, etc.
> (Levi-Strauss: 1968, p.295)

Levi-Strauss's approach was not very
satisfying. The Jane Eagle Hospital was more than
the sum of its different cultural parts. It had
its own distinct identity and its own history. It
was a physically bounded unit. For the patients
and for some members of the staff, especially the
nurses who lived on the hospital estate, the
hospital was the centre of their life. They had
few or no relationships with individuals outside
the hospital and spent most of their time inside
the hospital. Some nurses from overseas
(approximately 30% of the nurses were from
overseas) had little experience of English life
outside the hospital. The hospital culture
involved a distinctive way of grouping,
classifying and talking about patients.

Anthropologists, who take or seek a holistic
rather than a pluralistic definition of culture,
would reject Levi-Strauss's approach and would
seek the distinctive and defining characteristics
of culture. They would often find this distinctive
characteristic in the language of a group. The
profound ties between language and culture
underlie the Sapir-Whorf hypothesis which is based
on the belief that language not only facilitates
the transmission of culture but actually creates
it, by shaping the way in which members of a

language group perceive the world. Sapir summarised his position in the following way:

> Human beings do not live in the objective
> world alone, nor alone in the world of
> social activity as ordinarily understood,
> but are very much at the mercy of the
> particular language which has become the
> medium of expression for their society...
> The fact of the matter is that the "real
> world" is to a large extent unconsciously
> built upon the language habits of the
> group. No two languages are ever
> sufficiently similar to be considered as
> representing the same social reality. The
> worlds in which different societies live
> are distinct worlds, not merely the same
> world with different labels attached.
> (Sapir: 1929, p.209)

Ethnoscientists, following a similar logic, have given primacy to the cognitive aspects of culture. The evidence for these cognitive aspects has usually been derived from the language of a group, especially the ways in which the group names kin etc. For example, Goodenough has defined culture in the following way:

> culture is not a material phenomenon; it
> does not consist of things, people,
> behavior or emotions. It is rather
> an organization of these things. It is
> the forms of things that people have in
> mind, their models for perceiving,
> relating, and otherwise interpreting
> them. (Goodenough: 1964, p.36)

However the relationship between the boundary of a language and the boundary of a culture is clearly not a simple one to one relationship of concordance. In nonindustrial societies, there is frequently a wide diversity of languages and there are areas, often relatively small areas, inhabited by groups who speak different languages but who appear to share many customs, practices etc. (Bright and Bright: 1965). In the study of industrial societies, a different problem is encountered. Improvements in communications, especially the development of the mass media, have resulted in an increasing homogeneity of language.

Conclusion

For example English is not only the first language
of most of the citizens of Great Britain,
Ireland, the U.S.A. and countries of the "Old
Commonwealth" but is also used as a language in
many countries in the "New Commonwealth". It has
also become a major international language.

Although these different groups use the same
language, they use this language in different
ways. Words can be given different meanings
according to the cultural context in which they
are used. A dictionary attempts to provide a
"standard" meaning for a word and the specific
meaning it may acquire in some contexts but it
cannot list all the contexts and all the meanings.
For example it is possible to contrast the
dictionary definitions of "grade" and the meaning
it had for nurses at the Jane Eagle Hospital. The
Oxford English Dictionary gives the following
definitions of grade:

1. (in Mathematics) A degree; the 90th
   part of a right angle as a quadrant.

2. A step or stage in a process; rarely
   specifically a step in preferment.

3. A degree in the scale of rank, dignity,
   proficiency, etc.; a number of persons
   holding the same position in the scale;
   a class.

4. A degree of comparative quality of
   value; a class of things of the same
   quality or value.

5. (in Pathology) Degree or intensity (of
   a disease).

6. A result of cross-breeding, a hybrid.

7. (in Zoology) A group of animals
   presumed to have branched from the
   common stem at about the same point of
   its development.

8. (in Philology) The position occupied in
   an ablaut-series by a particular vowel
   or form of a root.

9. (in the English of the U.S.A.)

        a. Gradient. b. An inclined position of railway or road. c. (U.S. locally) In mining districts: A portion of road.

10. Of a surface: Degree of altitude; level (rare). (The Shorter Oxford Dictionary: 1969, pp.817-818)

The meaning of "grade" at the Jane Eagle was obviously related to the dictionary definition, but the dictionary did not cover the full meaning of the term nor could it show the importance of the concept at the Jane Eagle Hospital.

"Grade" was one of the key concepts at the hospital which was especially important to a grasp of the Jane Eagle culture. Other cultures also have key concepts. For example Geertz has described the importance of cock fighting in Bali (Geertz: 1973) and Evans-Pritchard the importance of cattle for the Nuer. Evans-Pritchard suggested that it was not possible to understand the Nuer, if the observer did not understand the importance of cattle in their culture:

> it is not possible to discuss with Nuer their daily affairs, social connexions, ritual acts, or, indeed any subject, without reference to cattle which are the core round which daily life is organized and the medium through which social and mystical relations are expressed ... The over-emphasis on cattle, whatever be the subject of speech, continually focuses attention on them and makes them the superlative value of Nuer life. (Evans-Pritchard: 1940, p.48)

Thus in most cultures there are central concepts and dominant symbols. These stand out as pervasive and important as a means of characterising the culture and providing a way of grasping the culture and its values.

At the Jane Eagle Hospital the patients formed this cultural focus. They were the main focus of interest and provided the main topic for conversation and discussion. The classifications and the special terminologies were all concerned with organising and describing the patients. Just as a study of the ecological setting and system of

Conclusion

production of the Nuer provides only a partial
explanation of importance of cattle in Nuer
culture (it does not fully explain the symbolism
of and mystical association of cattle), so the
institutional setting of the hospital, especially
its socio-legal context and its specific duties to
care for and control one type of dependant,
provides only a partial explanation of the
importance and centrality of the patients in the
hospital culture.

   The relationship between sub-cultures and
distinctive styles of language use is a well
established phenomenon in industrial societies.
Occupational groups have their own jargon,
minority groups have their own slang and deviant
groups such as drug addicts, have developed
vocabularies that allow them to openly discuss
deviant acts. These "languages" are closely
related to group identity and group membership and
an aspiring member of the group has to learn to
speak their "language" properly before he or she
is accepted as a full group member. Bernstein
(1973) and Douglas have both examined the relation
between speech and group identity. Bernstein has
contrasted restricted codes in which the language
of a speaker is closely, indeed inseparably,
enmeshed with his or her group identity, with
elaborated codes, in which the language of a
speaker and his or her group identity are clearly
separated. Douglas described the two codes in the
following way:

      The restricted code is deeply enmeshed in
         the immediate social structure,
         utterances have a double purpose: they
         convey information, yes, but they also
         express the social structure, embellish
         and reinforce it. The second function
         is the dominant one, whereas the
         elaborated code emerges as a form of
         speech which is progressively more and
         more free of the second function.
         (Douglas: 1970, p.23)

   The use of grade terminology can be seen as a
form of restricted code. When a nurse described a
patient as "low grade", the nurse was not only
providing, in a shorthand form, information about
the patient but was also defining himself or
herself and the audience as competent members of

245

the hospital culture.

However context was important in another way. The difference between context dependent and context independent codes is similar to Bourdieu's distinction between context dependent practice and context free theory (Bourdieu: 1977, pp.16-22). The formal interviewing methods, which I used were based on this theoretical discourse and therefore tended to produce a context free model of the hospital such as the one produced by Jones and her team. However the context had to be reestablished through observation of and participation in practice.

At the Jane Eagle Hospital the patients formed the central focus of staff interest and there was a distinctive set of terms to describe the patients. The most important and distinctive set were those associated with the classification of wards; "low grade", "high grade" and "cot and chair". These terms were not only used as labels for groups of wards, they also had a whole range of meanings and associations attached to them. For example the term "cot and chair" signified high dependency. Patients labelled in this way were seen as physically vulnerable and relatively passive.

However the typifications associated with the terms did not exhaust their meaning. There were also analogies associated with these terms. For example "cot and chair" patients were sometimes referred to as "vegetables". These analogies enabled the nurses to develop the meaning of the main grade classification. However it was important to study these analogies within the context of the hospital, as the terms were used metaphorically and not in their strict dictionary sense. It was easy to misjudge the sense in which nurses meant these analogies. For example the term "child" was used to describe all the hospital patients as well as one category within that group, usually the "high grade" patients but occasionally "low grades" were contrasted to "high grades" as "children" to "adults".

These organic analogies provided the staff with a way of talking about a phenomenon that was both difficult to understand and discuss, human beings who lacked many of the distinctive characteristics of that class. The analogies provided an integrated and comprehensive framework that related different groups of patients to each other and to normality.

Thus in the second part of the book, I was able to show that the grade classification provided nurses and other members of staff with an integrated and comprehensive view of the patients. This view I presented as being the distinctive and central concern of the hospital staff.

9.4 THE HOSPITAL: IDEAS AND ACTIONS

A third theme in this book has been the relationship between ideas and actions. In the second part of the book, I examined the classifications of the patients by the hospital staff as systems of ideas about the nature of the patients. In the third part of the book, I examined the ways in which these ideas influenced staff actions.

A major theme in sociology has been the influence of norms on social actions. Although norms have been defined in a variety of ways, they are usually seen as the generally accepted pattern of behaviour in a social group. In Parsons's analysis of the social systems of industrial society, norms play a key role in cultural tradition which he defined as a shared symbolic system integrated with socially prescribed actions:

> A symbolic system of meanings is an
> element of order "imposed" as it were
> on the realistic situation ... the
> mutuality of expectations is oriented
> on the shared order of symbolic
> meanings ... The orientation to a
> normative order, and the mutual
> interlocking of expectations and
> sanctions which will be fundamental
> to our analysis of social systems
> is rooted, therefore, in the deepest
> fundamentals of the action frame of
> reference. (Emphasis in the original
> text) (Parsons: 1951, pp.11-12)

Parsons also extended his analysis of norms to illness and disease. He identified a special sick role which ill people could occupy and defined it as conditionally legitimated deviance (Parsons: 1951, pp.205-244).

The concept of disease as conditionally

legitimated deviance has been developed by Freidson, who examined the ways in which, and the degrees to which, the social deviance implicit in illness is legitimated, and by Fabrega who focused on the different norms involved. For example Fabrega defined disease in the following way:

> I submit that as generally used by social scientists, physicians, and lay persons as well, the term disease appears to signify a person-centred undesirable deviation or discontinuity in the value of one or more of any number of different measures that can characterize an individual through time (emphasis in the original text). (Fabrega: 1974, p.125)

I could have analysed the material recorded in this book in terms of norms. Using this approach the ideas associated with the patient classification system would have provided the normative base for the activities observed. Indeed there would have been a reasonable fit between the ideas recorded in the second part of this book and the activities recorded in the third part. If the analysis of meal times is used as example, then the classification of patients could be interpreted as providing prescriptive norms for the overall pattern of staff/patient relations on the three wards and for the specific pattern of staff/patient relations during mealtimes. At the overall level the normative prescription for high grade patients would be a homely environment and a relaxed routine; for low grade patients a tough environment and a rigid routine and for cot and chair patients there could be no defined environment or ward routine. At the specific level of meal the following normative prescriptions could be derived, meals on cot and chair wards were to be organised as routine body servicing, meals on low grade wards were to be organised like animal feeding times and meals on high grade wards were to provide for the social development of patients and were to be more like social events.
However I found this an unsatisfactory explanation for the actions I observed. This approach would have explained some but not all the activities I observed. It would have explained the fact of variation between the three wards but

Conclusion

it could not have explained the precise form this variation took. When I examined the management of individual patients, the relationship between norms and actions was even more problematic. In all three cases staff recognised the individuality of the patient and therefore the need to apply the "rules" in a special way. If the normative approach was adopted the different explanations and circumstances of the patients and the different "rules" they broke should have resulted in different modes of control. However I could find little relationship between the methods of control used by nurses and the different explanations. Nurses used routine methods of control that seemed to have little regard to the circumstances of each case. The control was concerned with the maintenance of status rather than the breach of any specific rule. The rules did not cause the control, they justified it.

The emphasis on norms and rules has been subject to critical comment. Crime and law breaking have been central to the study of deviance and norms. Studies of crime have suggested that the context of law breaking and the relative status of participants has an important part to play in the consequences and social meaning ascribed to breach of rules. A breach of the rules is only classified as a deviance in certain circumstances. Cicourel has suggested that the attitudes of law enforcement agents play a key role in determining which breaches are defined as crime and which are not:

> When the police discover or are called to
> the scene of a supposed violation of the
> legal order, their sense of social
> structure and memory of past events in
> the neighborhood provide initial
> interpretations as to what happened.
> (Cicourel: 1976, p.328)

The importance of status and social context is also evident in the reaction to mental illness (Hollingshead and Redlich: 1958) and death (Glaser and Strauss: 1965).

Bourdieu has pushed the criticism of rules and norms a stage further. Cicourel's analysis maintained the importance of norms. For Cicourel they were an important factor in explaining observed behaviour, albeit not the only factor.

Conclusion

However Bourdieu has suggested that the use of the
concept of rules in the analysis of some cultures
is not just inadequate but also misleading:

> in social formations where, as in Kabylia
> (Algeria), there exists no judicial
> apparatus endowed with a monopoly of
> physical or even symbolic violence
> and where clan assemblies function as
> simple arbitration tribunals, that is,
> as more or less expanded family councils,
> the rules of customary laws have some
> practical efficacy only to the extent
> that, skilfully manipulated by the
> holders of authority within the clan
> (the "guarantors"), they "awaken", so
> to speak, the schemes of perception and
> appreciation deposited, in their
> incorporated state, in every member of
> the group, i.e. the dispositions of the
> habitus. (Bourdieu: 1977, p.17)

The rules existed in these cultures but they
were invoked to justify practical solutions whose
origins were in the practical strategies used by
actors in practical situations.

There were several points of similarity
between the situation I have described in this
book and that described by Bourdieu. In both
cases it was possible to identify practical
classifications, e.g. classification of time
amongst the Kabylia and classification of patients
at the Jane Eagle Hospital. Neither
classification was a description nor a set of
rules, rather both represented ways of talking
about the practical situation. Bourdieu's
discussion of the decontextualisation of usage
created by the graphic representation of time
amongst the Kabylia is equally applicable to
Jones's attempt to create a single integrated
model of the use of analogies in hospitals for the
mentally handicapped.

> The establishment of a single series thus
> creates ex nihilo a whole host of
> relations (of simultaneity, succession,
> or symmetry, for example) between terms
> and guide-marks of different levels,
> which, being produced and used in
> different situations, are never brought

> face to face in practice and thus
> compatible practically even when
> logically contradictory ... This
> (production of a synoptic diagram) makes
> it possible to apprehend at a glance,
> <u>uno intuitu et tota simul</u>, as Descartes
> said, <u>monothetically</u>, as Husserl put it,
> meanings which are produced and used
> polythetically, that is to say, not only
> one after another, but one by one, step
> by step. (Bourdieu: 1977, p.107)
> (Emphasis in the original text)

The situations in Bourdieu's case and at the Jane Eagle were also similar in that the same personalised modes of domination were used. However there was one important and crucial difference. Whereas the practical strategies in Kabylia showed considerable variation, those amongst the Jane Eagle nurses showed little variation. There was, in the words of one respondent, a "uniformity of response". Whereas there was considerable variation of status in Kabylia that allowed for ambiguity and variation in strategies, there was in the Jane Eagle Hospital very limited variation of status especially between the status of a member of staff and the status of a patient. The uniformity of strategies of control was based on the dominance of the members of staff.

Alaszewski, A.M. (1977) "Suggestions for the
     Reorganization of Nurse Training and
     Improvement of Patient Care in a Hospital
     for the Mentally Handicapped", Journal
     of Advanced Nursing, vol.2, pp.461-477.
Alaszewski, A.M. (1978a) "The Situation of
     Nursing Administrators in Hospitals for the
     Mentally Handicapped", Social Science and
     Medicine, Vol.12, pp.91-97.
Alaszewski, A.M. (1978b) "Problems in Measuring
     and Evaluating the Quality of Care in
     Mental Handicap Hospitals", Health and
     Social Service Journal, pp.A9-A15, 10 Mar.
Alaszewski, A.M. (1982) "Care Before Control",
     Health and Social Service Journal,
     pp.121-123, 28 Jan.
Alaszewski, A., Eccles, N. and Ong P. (1984)
     Measuring the Quality of Care:
     A Comparative Study of the Quality of
     Care of Mentally Handicapped Children
     in Long Stay Hospitals and in
     Dr. Barnardo's Intensive Support Unit,
     Discussion Paper No.2, Department of
     Social Policy and Professional Studies,
     University of Hull.
Allen, R.C. (1968) "Legal Norms and Practices
     Affecting the Mentally Deficient", in
     B.W. Richards, (ed) Proceedings of the
     First Congress of the International
     Association for the Scientific Study of
     Mental Deficiency, Jackson, Reigate.
Ayer, S. and Alaszewski, A. (1984) Community
     Care and the Mentally Handicapped:
     Services for Mothers and their Mentally
     Handicapped Children, Croom Helm.

Bibliography

Barth, F. (1966) Models of Social Organization, Royal Anthropological Institute, Occasional Paper 23.

Becker, H.S. (1958) "Problems of Inference and Proof in Participant Observation", American Sociological Review, Vol.23, pp.652-660.

Becker, H.S. (1963) Outsiders : Studies in the Sociology of Deviance, New York, The Free Press.

Belknap, I. (1956) Human Problems of a State Mental Hospital, New York, McGraw-Hill.

Bernstein, B. (1973) Class, Codes and Control, Vol.1 : Theoretical Studies Towards a Sociology of Language, Paladin.

Bettelheim, B. (1959) "Feral Children and Autistic Children", The American Journal of Sociology, Vol.64, pp.455-467.

Bourdieu, P. (1977) Outline of a Theory of Practice, trans. by R. Nice, Cambridge, Cambridge University Press.

Bloch, M. (1977) "The Past and the Present in the Present", Man, New Series, Vol.12, pp.278-292.

Boswell, D. (1977) "Sociological Study of the Residential Care of Mentally Handicapped Adults", unpublished Ph.D. thesis, University of Manchester.

Bourdillon, M.F.C. (1978) "Knowing the World or Hiding It : A Response to Maurice Bloch", Man, New Series, Vol.13, pp.591-599.

Bright, J.O., and Bright, W. (1965) "Semantic Structures in North-Western California and the Sapir-Whorf Hypothesis", in E.A. Hammel, (ed) "Formal Semantic Analysis" American Anthropologist, Vol.67.

Brown, G.W., (1975) "The Mental Hospital as an Institution", Social Science and Medicine, Vol.7, pp.407-424.

Bulmer, M. (ed) (1977) Sociological Research Methods : an Introduction, Macmillan.

Bulmer, R. (1967) "Why is the Cassowary not a Bird? A Problem of Zoological Taxonomy among the Karam of the New Guinea Highlands", Man, New Series, Vol.2, pp.5-25.

Bury, M. (1974) "Life on Yellow Ward", New Society, 2 May, pp.249-250.

Caudill, W.A. (1958) The Psychiatric Hospital as a Small Society, Cambridge, Mass., Harvard University Press.

Bibliography

Cicourel, A.V. (1964)   Method and Measurement in
    Sociology, New York,The Free Press.
Cicourel, A.V. (1976)   The Social Organization of
    Juvenile Justice, Heinemann.
Cohen, S. and Taylor, L. (1977)   "Talking about
    Prison Blues", in C. Bell and H. Newby
    (eds.) Doing Sociological Research, George
    Allen and Unwin.
Commissioners in Lunacy (1914) 68th Report,
    H.M.S.O.
Cooper, J.E. (1972) Psychiatric Diagnosis in New
    York and London, Oxford University Press.
Coser, R.L. (1963)   "Alienation and the Social
    Structure" in E. Freidson, (ed)
    The Hospital in Modern Society, New York,
    The Free Press.
Culyer, A.J. (1976)   Need and the National Health
    Service, Martin Robertson.
Dartington, T., Jones, P., Hilgerdorf, L. and
    Irving, B., (1973) "Balderton Hospital -
    The Nursing Perspective", in T. Dartington,
    P. Jones, L. Hilgerdorf and B. Irving,
    Balderton Hospital Research Project, The
    Tavistock Institute of Human Relations.
Dendy, M. (1920) "On the Training and Management
    of Feeble-Minded Children" in C.P. Lapage,
    Feeble-Mindedness in Children of School-Age,
    Manchester, The University Press.
D.H.S.S. (1971) Better Services for the
    Mentally Handicapped, Cmnd. 4683, H.M.S.O..
D.H.S.S. (1972) Census of Mentally Handicapped
    Patients in Hospitals in England and Wales,
    Statistical and Research Report Series,
    No.3, H.M.S.O..
D.H.S.S. (1976) Personnel, Staff Training,
    Proposals on Aspects of the Briggs Report
    on Nursing, H.M.S.O..
D.H.S.S. (1980) Mental Handicap: Progress,
    Problems and Priorities, D.H.S.S..
D.H.S.S. (1981) Press Release, Mental
    Handicap - Priorities for the 1980's,
    81/272, D.H.S.S..
D.H.S.S. (1983) Press Release, Norman Fowler
    Opens Homes for Severely Mentally
    Handicapped - Government Cash
    for Dr. Barnardo's Scheme, D.H.S.S..
Douglas, M. (1966) Purity and Danger, Routledge
    and Kegan Paul.
Douglas, M. (1970) Natural Symbols, Barrie and
    Rockliff.

Bibliography

Douglas, M. (1975) _Implicit Meanings_, Routledge
   and Kegan Paul.
Dugdale, R.L. (1910) _The Jukes : A Study in_
   Crime, Disease and Heredity, New York,
   Putnam (1st ed. 1877).
Dumont, L. (1965) "The Modern Conception of the
   Individual : Notes on Its Genesis and that
   of Concomitant Institutions", _Contributions_
   to Indian Sociology, Vol.8, pp.13-61.
Dumont, L. (1970) _Homo Hierarchicus_, trans. by
   M. Salisbury, Weidenfeld and Nicolson.
Durkheim, E. and Mauss, M. (1969) _Primitive_
   Classification, trans. by R. Needham,
   Cohen and West.
Edgerton, R.B. (1967) _The Cloak of Competence_,
   Berkeley, Calif., University of California
   Press.
Evans-Pritchard, E.E. (1937) _Witchcraft, Oracles_
   and Magic among the Azande, Oxford at the
   Clarendon Press.
Evans-Pritchard, E.E. (1940) _The Nuer_, Oxford at
   the Clarendon Press.
Evans-Pritchard, E.E. (1956) _Nuer Religion_,
   Oxford at the Clarendon Press.
Fabrega, H. (1974) _Disease and Social Behavior_,
   Cambridge, Mass., The M.I.T. Press.
Firth, R. (1961) _Elements of Social Organization_,
   Watts.
Flynn, R.J. and Nitsch, K.E. (eds.) (1980)
   Normalization, Social Integration
   and Community Services, Baltimore,
   University Park Press.
Foucault, M. (1967) _Madness and Civilization_,
   trans. by R. Howard, Tavistock.
Frake, C.O. (1961) "The Diagnosis of Disease
   among the Subanun of Mindanao", _American_
   Anthropologist, Vol.63, pp.113-132.
Freidson, E. (1975) _Profession of Medicine_,
   New York, Dodd, Mead and Co.
Galton, F. (1869) _Hereditary Genius_, Macmillan.
Geertz, C. (1973) _The Interpretation of Cultures_,
   New York, Basic Books.
Glaser, B.G. and Strauss, A.L. (1965), _Awareness_
   of Dying, Chicago, Ill., Aldine.
Glaser, B.G. and Strauss, A.L. (1967) _The_
   Discovery of Grounded Theory, Weidenfeld and
   Nicolson.
Goddard, H.L. (1931) _The Kallikak Family_, New
   York, Macmillan, 1931, (1st ed. 1912).
Goffman, E. (1968) _Asylums_, Penguin.

Goodenough, W.H. (1964) "Cultural Anthropology and Linguistics", in D.H. Hymes (ed), Language in Culture and Society, New York, Harper and Row.

Goody, J. (1977) The Domestication of the Savage Mind, Cambridge, Cambridge University Press, 1977.

Greer, S.A. (1969) The Logic of Social Inquiry, Chicago, Ill., Aldine.

Gunzberg, H.C. (1968) "The Assessment and Evaluation of Mentally Handicapped Children", in B.W. Richards (ed) Proceedings of the First Congress of the International Association for the Scientific Study of Mental Deficiency, Reigate, Jackson.

Hales, A. (1978) The Children of Skylark Ward, Cambridge, Cambridge University Press.

Halliday, M.A.K. (1961) "Categories of the theory of grammar", World, Journal of the Linguistic Circle of New York, Vol.17, pp.241-291.

Hammel, E.A. (1969) "Formal Semantic Analysis", American Anthropogist, Special Publication, Vol. 67, pp.1-316.

Harris, A.I. with Cox, E. and Smith, C.R.W. (1971) Handicapped and Impaired in Great Britain, H.M.S.O..

Harris, M. (1964) The Nature of Cultural Things, New York, Random House.

Hassell, D. (1971) "Patient Dependency related to Nurse Staffing in M.S. Hospital", Nursing Times, pp.77-80and pp.83-84, 20 May and 27 May.

Hay, J.R. (1975) The Origins of the Liberal Welfare Reforms: 1906-1914, Macmillan.

Hindess, B. (1973) The Use of Official Statistics in Sociology, MacMillan.

Hindess, B. (1977) Philosophy and Methodology in the Social Sciences, Harvester.

Hollingshead, A. and Redlich, F.C. (1958) Social Class and Mental Illness, New York, Wiley.

Howe, S.G. (1976) "Report of Commission to inquire into the conditions of idiots of the Commonwealth of Massachusetts" (1st published 1848) reprinted in M. Rosen, G.R. Clark and M.S. Kivitz (eds.) The History of Mental Retardation: Volume 1 Baltimore, University Park Press.

Hunter, R. and MacAlpine, I. (1974) Psychiatry

for the Poor : 1851 Colney Hatch - Friern
Hospital 1973, Dawsons.

Jones, K. (1972) A History of the Mental Health
Service, Routledge and Kegan Paul.

Jones, K. (1975) Opening the Door, Routledge
and Kegan Paul.

Jones, K. and Fowles, A.J. (1984) Ideas on
Institutions: Analysing the Literature
on Long-Term Care and Custody, Routledge
and Kegan Paul.

Jones, K. and Sidebotham R. (1962) Mental
Hospitals at Work, Routledge and Kegan
Paul.

Kanner, L. (1964) A History of the Care and
Study of the Mentally Retarded, Springfield,
Ill., C.C. Thomas.

Kendall, A. and Moss, P. (1972) Intergration or
Segregation? Campaign for the Mentally
Handicapped

King, R.D., Raynes, N.V. and Tizard, J. (1971)
Patterns of Residential Care, Routledge and
Kegan Paul.

Kushlick, A. (1967) "A Method of Evaluating the
Effectiveness of a Community Health
Service" Social and Economic Administration,
Vol.1, pp.29-48.

Kushlick, A. (1968) "The Wessex Plan for
Evaluating the Effectiveness of Residential
Care for the Severely Subnormal", in B.W.
Richards (ed) Proceedings of the First
Congress of the International Association
for the Scientific Study of Mental
Deficiency, Reigate, Jackson.

Kushlick, A. (1974) "The Need for Residential
Care : The Wessex Experiment" in
H.C. Gunzburg (ed) Experiments in the
Rehabilitation of the Mentally Handicapped,
Butterworths.

Kushlick, A., Blunden, R. and Cox, G., (1973)
"A Method of Rating Behaviour
Characteristics for Use in Large
Scale Surveys of Mental Handicap",
Psychological Medicine, Vol.3, pp.466-478.

Laslett, P. (1965) The World we have Lost,
Methuen.

Leach, E. (1976) Culture and Communication,
Cambridge, Cambridge University Press.

Leach, R.A. (1913) The Mental Deficiency Act,
1913, The Local Goverment Press.

Levi-Strauss, C. (1963) Totemism, trans. by

Bibliography

R. Needham, Pelican.

Levi-Strauss, C. (1968) Structural Anthropology, trans. by C. Jacobson and B.G. Schoepf, Allen Lane.

Levi-Strauss, C. (1969) The Elementary Structures of Kinship, trans. by J.H. Bell, J.R. von Sturmer and R. Needham, Eyre and Spottiswoode.

Levi-Strauss, C. (1970) The Raw and the Cooked, trans. by J. Weightman and D. Weightman Cape, 1970.

Levi-Strauss, C. (1972) The Savage Mind, Weidenfeld and Nicolson.

Levy-Bruhl, L. (1910) Les Fonctions Mentales, Paris, Alcen.

Lockett, R.W. (1972) "Assessment of Patients' Dependency", Nursing Times, Occasional Paper, 13 Apr., pp.57-60.

Lomax, M. (1921) The Experiences of an Asylum Doctor, Allen and Unwin.

Lukes, S. (1974) Power : A Radical View, Macmillan.

Lyle, J.G. (1960) "The Effect of an Institutional Environment upon the Verbal Development of Imbecile Children, III, The Brooklands Residential Family Unit", Journal of Mental Deficiency Research, Vol.4, pp.14-23.

MacAndrew, C. and Edgerton, R. (1964) "The Everyday Life of Institutionalised Idiots", Human Organization, Vol.23, pp.312-8.

McKinlay, J.B. (1975) "Clients and Organizations" in J.B. McKinlay (ed) Processing People: Cases in Organizational Behaviour, New York, Holt, Rinehart and Winston.

Maine, H.J.S. (1866) Ancient Law, John Murray (3rd ed).

Malson, L. (1972) Wolf Children with the Wild Boy of Aveyron by Jean Itard, New Left Books.

Mauss, M. (1979a) Seasonal Variations of the Eskimo: A Study of the Social Morphology, trans. by J.J.Fox, Routledge and Kegan Paul.

Mauss, M. (1979b) Sociology and Psychology, Essays, trans. by B. Brewster, Routledge and Kegan Paul.

Mental Deficiency Act (1913) 3 and 4, George 5, C.28.

Menzies, I.E.P. (1960) "A Case Study in the

Bibliography

Functioning of Social Systems as a Defense against Anxiety", Human Relations, Vol.13, pp.95-121.

Mercer, J.R. (1965) "Social System Perspective and Clinical Perspective", Social Problems, Vol.13, pp.18-34.

Mercer, J.R. (1968) "Labeling the Mentally Retarded", in E. Rubington and M.S. Weinberg (eds.) Deviance : The Interactionist Perspective, New York, Macmillan.

Mercer, J.R. (1973) Labeling the Mentally Retarded, Berkeley, Calif., University of California Press.

Metzger, D. and Williams, G. (1963a) "Tenejapa Medicine, 1, The Curer", South-Western Journal of Anthropology, Vol.19, pp.216-234.

Metzger, D. and Williams, G. (1963b) "A Formal Ethnographic Analysis of Tenejapa Ladino Weddings", American Anthropologist, Vol.65, pp.1076-1101.

Miller, E.J. and Gwynne, G.V. (1972) A Life Apart, Tavistock.

Morris, P. (1969) Put Away, Routledge and Kegan Paul.

Nadel, S.F. (1951) The Foundations of Social Anthropology, Cohen and West.

National Health Service (1972) Annual Report of the Hospital Advisory Service ... for the Year 1971, H.M.S.O..

Needham, R. (ed) (1971) Rethinking Kinship and Marriage, Tavistock.

Newby, H. (1977) "In the Field : Reflections on the Study of Suffolk Farm Workers", in C. Bell and H. Newby (eds.) Doing Sociological Research, George Allen and Unwin.

Ong, B.N. and Alaszewski A. (1984) The Training of Staff for the Intensive Support Unit for Profoundly Mentally Handicapped Children, Working Paper No.1, Institute for Health Studies, University of Hull.

Oswin, M. (1971) The Empty Hours, Penguin.

Parsons, T. (1951) The Social System, Routledge and Kegan Paul.

Radcliffe-Brown, A.R. (1952) Structure and Function in Primitive Society, Cohen and West.

Rapaport, R.N. (1960) Community as Doctor, Tavistock.

Bibliography

Report from the Committee of the House of
    Commons on Madhouses in England (1815)
    Baldwin, Cradock and Joy.
Report of the Committee of Enquiry into Mental
    Handicap Nursing and Care (1979)   Chairman
    Peggy Jay, Vol.I, Cmnd. 7468-1, H.M.S.O..
Report of the Committee of Inquiry into
    Allegations of Ill-treatment of Patients and
    Other Irregularities at the Ely Hospital,
    Cardiff (1969) Cmnd. 3975, H.M.S.O..
Report of the Committee of Inquiry into
    Normansfield Hospital (1978)   Cmnd. 7357,
    H.M.S.O..
Report of the Department Committee appointed by
    the Board of Control with the approval of
    the Minister of Health to consider matters
    relating to the Construction of Colonies
    for Mental Defectives (1931) H.M.S.O..
Report of the Departmental Committee on
    Sterilization (1934) Cmd. 4483, Chairman
    L.G. Brock, H.M.S.O..
Report of the Mental Deficiency Committee, being
    a Joint Committee of the Board of
    Education and the Board of Control (1929)
    Chairman A. Wood, H.M.S.O..
Report of the Royal Commission on the Care and
    Control of the Feeble Minded (1908)
    Cd. 420, H.M.S.O..
Rooff, M. (1957) Voluntary Societies and Social
    Policy, Routledge and Kegan Paul.
Rosengren, W.R. and DeVault, S. (1963) "The
    Sociology of Time and Space in an
    Obstetrical Hospital", in E. Freidson (ed)
    The Hospital in Modern Society, New York,
    The Free Press.
Roth, J.A. (1957) "Ritual and Magic in the
    Control of Contagion", American Sociological
    Review, Vol.22, pp.310-314.
Rothman, D.J. (1971) The Discovery of the Asylum
    Boston, Mass., Little, Brown and Co.
Rothman, D.J. (1980) Conscience and Convenience:
    The Asylum and its Alternatives in
    Progressive America, Little, Brown and
    Company, Boston.
Ryan, J. (1972) "I.Q. : The Illusion of
    Objectivity", in K. Richardson, D. Spears
    and M. Richards (eds.) Race, Culture and
    Intelligence, Penguin.
Ryan, J. (1976) "The Production and Management
    of Stupidity", in M. Wadsworth and

D. Robinson (eds.) <u>Studies in Everyday</u>
<u>Medical Life</u>, Martin Robertson.

Sapir, E. (1929) "The Status of Linguistics as
a Science", <u>Language</u>, Vol.5, pp.207-214.

Schroyer, T. (1971) "The Critical Theory of Late
Capitalism", in G. Fischer (ed)
<u>The Revival of American Socialism</u>
New York, Oxford University Press.

Schutz, A (1971) <u>Collected Paper, 1,</u>
<u>The Problems of Social Reality</u>, The Hague,
Nijhoff.

Scull,A.T. (1979) <u>Museums of Madness : The Social</u>
<u>Organization of Insanity in Nineteenth-</u>
<u>Century England</u>, Allen Lane.

<u>The Shorter Oxford English Dictionary</u> (1969)
prepared by W. Little, H.W. Fowler and
J. Coulson, revised and edited by
C.T. Onions, Oxford at the Clarendon Press,
3rd ed.

Silverman, D. (1970) <u>The Theory of Organisations</u>,
Heinemann.

Silverman, D. (1975) "Accounts of
Organizations", in McKinlay, J.B. (ed)
<u>Processing People</u>, New York, Holt, Rinehart
and Winston.

Smith, B.C. (1976) <u>Policy Making in British</u>
<u>Government</u>, Martin Robertson.

Stanton, A.H. and Schwartz, M.J. (1954)
<u>The Mental Hospital</u>, New York, Basic
Books.

Stark, L.R. (1969) "The Lexical Structure of
Quechua Body Parts", <u>Anthropological</u>
<u>Linguistics</u>, Vol.11, pp.1-5.

Strauss, A.L. et al., (1964) <u>Psychiatric</u>
<u>Ideologies and Institutions,</u>
The Free Press, New York.

Strauss, A.L. and Glaser, B.G. (1970) <u>Anguish :</u>
<u>A Case History of a Dying Trajectory</u>,
Martin Robertson.

Street, D., Vinter, R.D. and Perrow, C. (1966)
<u>Organization for Treatment</u>, New York,
The Free Press.

Tawney, R.H. (1931) <u>Equality</u>, Allen and Unwin.

Thomas, D., Firth, H. and Kendall. A. (1978)
<u>ENCOR , A Way Ahead</u>, Campaign for Mentally
Handicapped People

Tizard, J., Sinclair, I. and Clarke, R.V.G.
(1975) <u>Varieties of Residential</u>
<u>Experience</u>, Routledge and Kegan Paul.

Towell, D. (1975) <u>Understanding Psychiatric</u>

Nursing, Royal College of Nursing.

Towers, B.A. (1984) "The Management and Politics of a Public Expose: The Prestwich Inquiry of 1922", Journal of Social Policy, Vol.13, pp.41-61.

Townsend, P. (1962) The Last Refuge, Routledge and Kegan Paul.

Trist, E.L. et al. (1963) Organizational Choice, Tavistock.

Tuke, S. (1813) Description of the Retreat, An Institution near York, for Insane Persons of the Society of Friends, York,W. Alexander.

Tuke, S. (1964) Description of the Retreat, reprinted with an introd. by R. Hunter and I. MacAlpine, Dawsons.

Tylor, E.B. (1958) Origins of Culture, Volume 1, Gloucester, Mass., Smith, (1st ed. 1871).

Tyne, A. (1974) "Nursing Work and the Care of the Mentally Handicapped Patients" unpublished M.A. thesis, Department of Sociology, University of Essex.

Ullman   L.P. (1967)   Institution and Outcome, Oxford, Pergamon.

Voysey, M. (1975)   A Constant Burden, Routledge and Kegan Paul.

Weber, M. (1947)   The Theory of Social and Economic Organization, trans. by A.M. Henderson and T. Parsons, New York, The Free Press.

Whyte, W.F. (1955)   Street Corner Society, Chicago, Ill., University of Chicago Press.

Wing, J.K. and Brown, B.W. (1970) Institutionalism and Schizophrenia, Cambridge, Cambridge University Press.

Wolfensberger, W. (1974) The Origins and Nature of Institutions, Syracuse, New York, Syracuse University, Human Policy Press.

INDEX

SUBJECT INDEX

accounts 57, 75, 77-88
Adult Training Centre
  229
analogies 77, 85-6,
  246; adult 126, 131,
  134; animal 71-2,
  77, 112, 116,
  118-122, child
  77, 117, 119-121,
  126, 129-133; organic
  116-136; vegetable
  116-8, 120-1, 126,
  130, 132, 134, 185,
  246
anthropology (see
  social anthropology)
anti-institution 23-32
architecture 7-11, 26,
  33
asylum 8, 11, 23-4, 76
  103
autism 122

back ward (see ward)
Balderton Hospital
  77, 80
basic care 31-2, 65,
  153, 189, 234
Bethlem 7
block treatment 144
body servicing 158,
  172, 180-1, 248
brutality 38

Campaign for Mentally
  Handicapped People
  25
case conference 43,
  64, 91
classification 7,
  10-12, 19-21, 33-4
  46-7, 59;
  and anomalies 112-5;
  mixing patients 94-
  112; of wards 64-93;
clinical psychology 91,
  197-8
Colney Hatch 9-11
Colony (See mental
  deficiency colony)
community 25-6, 40, 77,
  86
consultant 42, 65,
  91-2, 96, 105, 196-7,
  208, 214, 220-2, 227
contract 5
culture 36, 40-49,
  52-4, 57, 59, 69, 75,
  123, 136, 143, 148,
  189, 240-7
cyclical time 189

Darenth Institutions 16
dayroom 37
decontextualisation
  131, 133-4, 250
dependency 5-7, 24-5,

263

Index

Index

Index

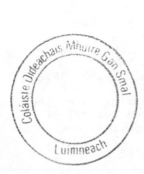